Why Your Doctor Can't Write

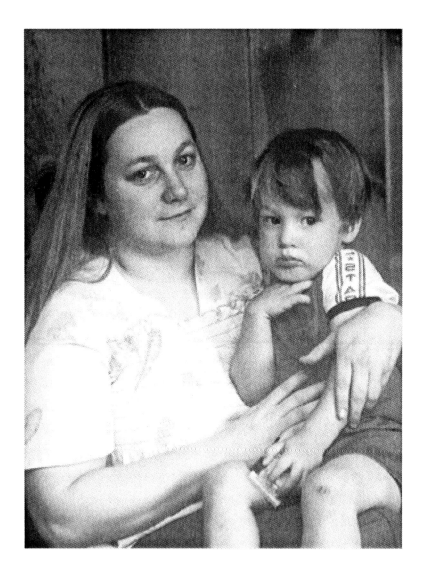

Bryan's mother holds him after he had his urinary tract enlarged. This urinary surgery was scheduled instead for a boy named Ryan.

Why Your Doctor Can't Write

Write

The Problem and a Solution

Donna Reid Connell Ed.D.

Writers Club Press

San Jose New York Lincoln Shanghai

Why Your Doctor Can't Write
The Problem and a Solution

Writers Club Press
an imprint of iUniverse.com, Inc.

For information address:
iUniverse.com, Inc.
620 North 48th Street, Suite 201
Lincoln, NE 68504-3467
www.iuniverse.com

ISBN: 0-595-13139-5

Printed in the United States of America

This book is dedicated to the memory and short life of Dr. William Crutcher, a most dedicated dermatologist. Bill had a passion for finding and eliminating deadly melanoma moles. Should you go to him for anything as simple as an itchy rash or warts on your hands Doctor Bill always looked further to be sure that melanoma was not hiding somewhere else on your body.

He did find one on a young woman accountant. But it was too late for her as the melanoma had already spread to her brain. After brain surgery she could no longer read and continue her career. Bill sent her to me for reading rehabilitation and volunteered to pay for her lessons.

His intense passion caused him to work such long hours that his own body finally wore out with a major heart attack at age 50. Like other doctors who have been taught to write in the archaic cursive form used in American schools both yesterday and today, his handwritten messages required a slow translation. A copy of one of his letters is in Chapter One. We miss you, Bill.

Physician, Do No Harm

From the Oath Taken
By All Doctors Today

CONTENTS

The Problem 1

Possible Causes of Illegibility 14

Can We Change? 43

Conclusion 89

Bibliography 95

Appendix 103

LIST OF ILLUSTRATIONS

Enlarged Diagnosis 7

Personal Note from a Physician 8

Hand Written Prescription 9

Prescriptions Written by German Physicians 9

Signatures of Well Known People 11

First Grade Letter 12

First Grade Letter 13

Syllable Writing 16

Profile Drawing 17

Oldest Known Alphabetic Graffiti 19

The Sinai Sphinx 20

Inscription Found in the Sinai 21

Greek Alphabet, 6th Century B.C. 23

Laubach's Phonetic English Language System 24

Classic Roman Capitals 26

Reproducing a Diamond Shape 27

Architect and Engineer Script 28

Roman Capitals Written Rapidly 29

Rapidly Written Capitals Today 30

How Capitals Became Simplified 31

From the Book of Kells 33

Chancery Cursive 35

Copperplate Cursive Capitals 36

Copperplate Lower Case 37

Standard School Cursive 37

Ball Stick Manuscript 40

School Cursive Capitals 41

Today's Reinvented Chancery Cursive 44

Modified Cursive Written on a Computer 45

D'Nealian Lower Case 46

D'Nealian Cursive 48

Italic Lower Case 50

Italic Written Rapidly 51

Chancery Capitals 52

Australian Lower Case 53

Beery-Butenika Scale 54

Alphabet Difficulty Scale 55

Capital Letter Difficulty 57

Ball Stick Difficulty 58

Italic Difficulty 59

D'Nealian Difficulty 60

Australian Difficulty 61

Simplified Lower Case
(monkey tails Removed, italic flat tops added) 62

Simplified Letters Grouped by Shape 64

Simplest Form in Continuous Communication 65

Japanese Language Symbols for Beginners 67

Nicolas, Age 3, Makes Vertical Lines 68

Tyler's Grocery List, Age 4 72

Tyler's Halloween Costume, Age 5 73

Tyler's Science Report 74

Emily's Story 78

Tyler's Signature 79

Efficient Grasp of Writing Tool 82

Primitive Infantile Tool Grip 83

Paper Position for Lefties 84

Kaci's Picture Story 86

Paul Uses Letters as Words and Syllables 87

Krista's Picture Story 88

About the Author 101

FOREWORD

Long ago, when I was a child at summer camp, it took a team of counselors and campers working together to decipher the postcards I received from my dad. He wasn't a doctor, but as a pharmacist deciphering prescriptions, I guess he thought that was how people were supposed to write.

Illegible handwriting can be dangerous. In this age of computers, American schools still teach handwriting the way it's been taught for the last three hundred years, except with much less frequency and intensity today. Donna Reid Connell, author and educator, has done extensive research into this issue and makes a compelling case for our need to upgrade instruction and change.

Dr. Barbara Nemko, Superintendent, Napa County Schools, California (February, 2000)

ACKNOWLEDGMENTS

To Dr. James M. Talcott, my orthopedist, who keeps my skeleton operating,

Dr. Roland Julis, my gerontologist, a specialist in the aging process, who keeps my insides functioning,

Dr. Robert E. Nasser, my opthalmologist, who helps me see,

Elly Pfau, M.A., my audiologist, who keeps my hearing aids operating,

Cynthia Ross, coach for my arthritis water exercise program,

Joan Watson, coach for my physical fitness program

Randy Goodrich, who solved my computer glitches and designed this book, and to

John Connell, my husband for 60 years who cooks and cares for my nutrition needs.

Were it not for these eight individuals, this book would not have been possible. In this last third of my life they have kept me thinking,

It's a Wonderful Life!

THE PROBLEM

Up to 98,000 Americans die every year, not from illness, birth defects, natural causes, or old age, but by unnecessary preventable mistakes! These deaths are not caused by fire, floods, earthquakes, hurricanes, or other natural disasters. They are not caused by terrorists dropping bombs on innocent victims. They are not caused by crashing of jumbo jets. Instead, in November, 1999, the Institute of Medicine, an arm of the National Academy of Sciences, reported that as many as 98,000 Americans die unnecessarily every year from medical mistakes made by physicians, pharmacists and other health care professionals.

In addition, the Department of Veterans' Affairs, in December, 1999, documented close to 3000 medical mistakes and mishaps in less than two years at veterans' hospitals throughout the country. More than 700 patients died in those cases.

The National Academy of Sciences report calls for a major overhaul of how the nation addresses medical errors. While other areas of the U.S. economy have coordinated safety programs that collect and analyze accident trends, there is not a centralized system to keep track of medical errors and use that information to prevent future mistakes. If such a system were put in place, the report predicts that the number of medical mistakes could be cut in half in five years. That still would leave 49,000 unnecessary deaths each year.

Responding to this disturbing report, President Clinton requested Congress to adopt a White House plan requiring hospitals nationwide to disclose serious and deadly mistakes. He also planned to order several new requirements that do not need congressional approval, including an immediate mandatory reporting requirement for the 500 Defense Department administered hospitals that serve an estimated 8 million people. In addition the Health Care Financing Administration will require error reduction plans this year in all 6000 hospitals that participate in Medicare.

The Food and Drug Administration has one year to develop new standards to help prevent medical mistakes caused by sound-alike drug names or look-alike products. The agency must also come up with new standards for labels that highlight common problems such as errors in dosage size.

The White House wants all hospitals to report errors within three years, but cannot force compliance without legislation from Congress. It sees its plan as a compromise between patient advocates who want full disclosure of medical mistakes and representatives of doctors and hospitals who fear more disclosure means more lawsuits. The White House wants a mandatory national reporting system, by hospital and by type of problem, administered by the states, that would collect information about preventable deaths and major injuries. Names of individual doctors or other health care workers would not be made public.

With the White House plan hospitals would not have to report less serious mistakes or close calls, but they hope that they would do so voluntarily. The plan states that the purpose is not to blame people or be punitive, but that the first step is to acknowledge our problem.

Several medical and public policy organizations have addressed this issue since the widely reported death of Boston Globe health columnist, Betsy Lehman, who died from a chemotherapy overdose in 1995. Part of the problem, according to the report, is that many new drugs have similar names, which are easily confused when orders are given by voice or are handwritten. Last year the Food and Drug Administration convinced a drug manufacturer to change the proposed name of a new arthritis drug from *Celebra to Celebrex. Celebra* was too easy to mistake for *Celesa* an antidepressant. But the new name can be mistaken for *Cerebyx,* a drug for epilepsy. Ads in medical journals from the makers of Celebrex warn doctors not to confuse this product with either *Cerebyx* or *Celesa.*

So far as is known about the thousands of fatalities by medical mistakes each year all of them have been caused by errors in communication. Errors include wrong diagnoses from mislabeled blood samples, mistaken treatments because of poorly labeled drugs, improper dosing because of faulty calculations and a simple lack of communication as a patient gets passed from one provider to the next. According to the Institute of Medicine report the most serious mistakes occur in busy settings such as emergency rooms and intensive care units.

These errors are not caused by uncaring doctors. Instead, a major part of the problem has been our confusing, inadequate and archaic handwriting instruction in both our public and private schools particularly during the last half of the 20th century. Several generations ago the curriculum of our education system was referred to as the three R's, *Reading, Riting and Rithmetic.* At that time it was common for school districts to have a handwriting specialist on their staffs.

Today the major components of academic achievement tests are Reading and Math. Occasionally a unit of Spelling is added by having students choose the correct form from a group of spellings. Writing, both composition and handwriting, are usually not tested. Some time ago I was involved in seeking a group of teachers to participate in a first-grade writing test. One teacher expressed a common attitude; *My class will be tested in Reading and Math. I cannot afford to spend any teaching time on Writing.*

Outdated instruction in handwriting today is directly related to the high numbers of medical errors. *Physician handwriting has traditionally not been something that has been looked upon highly by calligraphers,* said Peter Honig, who was deputy director of the Food and Drug Administration's office of post-marketing drug-risk assessment, the federal unit responsible for tracking medication errors.

Drs. Karen White and John Beary III of Georgetown University Hospital have shared their findings in the New England Journal of Medicine on the handwriting of 50 physicians as it appears on medical records. These doctors reported that a considerable portion of most handwritten medical records are illegible. Forty two of the reports on patients were not fully comprehensible. They concluded that, *The price we pay for illegibility includes lower quality of care, a waste of professional time, potential legal problems and a waste of resources in duplicating data.*

The handwriting problem is certainly not new. In 1980 officials at St. Elizabeth's Hospital in Belleville, Illinois, investigated an operating room mix-up in which a two-year-old boy named, Bryan, and a four-year-old boy named, Ryan, received surgery meant for each other. Bryan had his urinary tract enlarged. That procedure had been intended for Ryan, who, instead, had his tonsils and adenoids removed. After the error was discovered both youngsters received the operations for which they had been scheduled. The hospital administrator, Sister Paulette, apologized to the families and told them that they would not be billed for the second surgeries.

In a similar case in Philadelphia in 1979 two women at Graduate Hospital underwent at least partial operations for each other's maladies. The errors resulted in Ann Robinson mistakenly being cut open for back surgery and Virginia Edmonson mistakenly receiving a partial parathyroid operation. The Philadelphia health department, which investigated that mix-up, said the similar names of the two women (three syllables ending in *son*) caused the mix-ups of their charts.

Another case caused by misreading of patient's names occurred in New York in 1995 at the Memorial-Sloan Kettering Cancer Center. A neurosurgeon there operated on the wrong side of a patient's brain. He had confused the X-rays of two patients with unfamiliar Indian names. The patient receiving the wrong surgery did survive, but the operation left her with memory damage. In this case the neurosurgeon was fired. Subsequently he became chief of neurosurgery at Staten Island University Hospital where he was under state scrutiny following the death of another patient.

In 1995 in Miami surgeons amputated the wrong leg from a man whose diabetes had interfered with the circulation of his blood to the extent that amputation was necessary. At the same hospital a woman had arthroscopic surgery performed on the wrong knee. A few weeks later another disaster at this same hospital caused a man to die when he was *inappropriately removed from his ventilator because of mistaken identity.* When asked for a comment about these three incidents at one hospital, Dr. James S.Todd, who was serving at that time as the executive vice president of the American Medical Association, responded, *Unfortunately the rules established by the AMA and other protective agencies were not followed. What occurred in Florida was due to human failure. As for the physicians who get their licenses back, the AMA has no control. It is strictly up to the state licensing board to make the decisions.*

Few individuals would disagree that we do have a problem with adult handwriting in this country. It has been estimated that unreadable handwriting is annually costing the United States an astronomical number of dollars. The Post Office has reported that every year over a million pieces of mail end up in the dead letter office because of unreadable addresses. Over ten years ago they adopted a code using two capital letters for each state. To avoid California mail being missent to Colorado, Alaska mail being missent to Alabama, and Minnesota mail being missent to Massachusetts, or vice versa, we now are required to use capital letter codes for each state, such as *CA* and *CO, AK* and *AL* and *MN* and *MA.* And these must be made in carefully written block print capitals or the post office automatic sorting machines will reject and return them to sender.

Merchants report losses in the thousands of dollars because of the illegible sales slips written by their staff which has caused merchandise to be undeliverable. One of my college students expressed his concern about his part-time job. He was being promoted from warehouse duty to sales. *But, I can't write a sales slip so others can read it!* The National Geographic Society estimated that bad handwriting alone (not bad spelling) costs American businesses 70 million dollars a year in confusion, waste and ill will.

Similar to the post office attempt to solve illegible addresses, doctors have adopted a symbol system by reducing their handwriting to capital letter abbreviations. According to two Pennsylvania pharmacologists, one at Temple University and the other at Quakertown Community Hospital, thousands of these abbreviation codes for drugs and treatments can be misunderstood by those who carry out the physicians' orders. These pharmacologists publish a list of 600 medical abbreviations commonly used. In addition, they started the Medication Error Report Line which collects about 30 accounts of such blunders each month.

Everyone on the health team must be able to translate these abbreviation hieroglyphs. Too often they do not. Take, for instance the patient who required *PT*, the letter symbol for Prothrombin Time test which measures how long it takes the blood to clot. He was sent, instead, for Physical Therapy. Or consider the attendant who cleaned a patient's wound with TAB diet soda. The doctor's orders were for T.A.B., a triple antibiotic mixture.

The letters, *OS* in medical jargon stand for *left eye*. The letters *OJ* to the general public commonly represent orange juice. The letter *J* when written rapidly sometimes resembles an *S*. An attendant put potassium iodine solution in a patient's left eye instead of in his *OJ*. One instance not quite so disastrous was the order for three drops of an anesthetic and antibiotic in the right ear. The patient received an anal injection when the attendant translated the order to in the *R-ear*.

The letter, *U*, representing units, has been widely misread as *O* or sometimes *6*. When the letter, *U*, has not been written slowly and carefully beginning with a vertical line instead of a curve and showing an obvious opening at the top, the abbreviation *IU* for one unit has been misread as the number *10*. This error has been responsible for a number of fatal overdoses in which ten times the prescribed amount of drug has been given.

The published list of medical abbreviations grows daily as new drugs come on the market and medical treatments are developed or refined.

In an attempt to produce doctors who relate better to patients, the Association of American Medical Colleges announced in 1989 an overhaul of its medical school admission test. The aim was to make it less technical and to stress oral and written communication skills. The revised test includes four sections: biological sciences, physical sciences, verbal reasoning and writing essays. The intent of the components of verbal reasoning and essay writing was to attract well-rounded candidates who can think logically and deal with patients as human beings. It was to improve the quality of patient care–what used to be called *bedside manner.* With the current universal use of computers in all levels of education it is doubtful that today's applicants for medical school have written an essay by hand since the sixth grade. It will be interesting to see if the Association of American Medical Colleges will continue to overhaul their entrance test to include handwriting.

Here is a copy of a diagnosis written by my own primary physician. Sometimes enlargement helps to decipher such illegible messages. In this case it does not seem to give much help.

Enlarged Diagnosis

Following is part of a note written to me by a dermatologist who was requesting that I give some basic reading lessons to one of his adult patients who had lost the ability to read after brain surgery for melanoma. Fortunately none of my reading treatments would be life threatening.

Personal Note from a Physician

Avandia, a diabetes drug, was prescribed on the next prescription. According to the Institute for Safe Medication practices it was mistaken for *coumadin* a blood thinner. The patient got only one dose before the doctor discovered the error. Notice that when the letter, *a*, is not slowly and carefully closed at the top it can be mistaken for the letter, *c*.

Hand Written Prescription

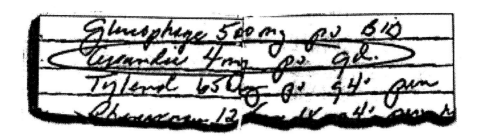

Illegibility is not particularly an American problem, but is common where other world cultures also still use the archaic joined cursive form of our alphabet which cannot be written rapidly and maintain legibility.

Prescriptions Written
by German Physicians

38304 Wolfenbüttel   Nr.10177

In an attempt to compensate for their illegible handwriting and prevent major medical mistakes some concerned doctors use an electronic voice recorder when making diagnoses which will then be translated and recorded by a medical secretary. Others hire a scribe to stand near them during diagnosis and write down what the doctor tells them.

Sometimes adults create a monogram of wriggly lines to stand for their signature, as if they were creating a logo to advertise themselves. One should not have to guess at what names these symbols stand for. Handwriting experts we call graphologists tell us that creative signatures like these are easiest to forge. Also, some individuals deliberately scrawl their name to cover up the evidence that they usually do not write it legibly.

Young students play the same game scrawling over a word they don't know how to spell, hoping the teacher won't observe it. Even kindergarten students, not sure of how to distinguish the letters, *d* and *b,* sometimes will invent a letter with a curve on both sides of the vertical line. This gives the reader a choice and these children avoid admitting they aren't sure of the distinction. Young students often ask me why people scrawl their own signatures like these that follow:

Signatures of Well Known People

Nancy Reagan

[George Bush signature]

[Henry Kissinger signature]

[O. J. Simpson signature]

John Lennon

[Donald Wayne signature]

Sigmund Freud

To share with his class, a student in one of my early primary classes brought a copy of a political message received by his parent in the mail. It was signed by George Bush, who was President at that time. When the other students saw his rapidly written illegible signature they decided to write to him to offer help in handwriting.

First Grade Letter

Dear President Bush,
    Your handwriting
is a little messy. I know
a way to make your hand
writing better. Write
slower. I am left handed too.
                    Your friend, Cole
            age 8

First Grade Letter

Dear President Bush,
   Your hand writing is not very good. You should get a tutor then you can write to us when you learn to write better. I'm left handed. If I can do it you can do it. I'm glad to help you.
   Love, Angelina   age 8

The president did not answer their letters.

POSSIBLE CAUSES OF ILLEGIBILITY

When confronted with their unreadable handwriting, doctors sometimes use the excuse that they lose their legibility in handwriting in medical training when they are forced to write so quickly to take copious notes in their classes. Do not graduate students in other professions also have to take many rapid notes during lectures?

More than likely there is something in the way students are originally taught to write or in the particular forms of letters they are usually taught in school which makes their writing illegible when written quickly. Illegible handwriting by American adults is to a great extent related to the two outdated forms of writing taught in most of our schools today, ball-stick manuscript and copperplate cursive.

A review of history tells us why these two commonly taught forms do not reflect our need for functional, simple, legible, unadorned, fluent handwriting that uses contemporary implements instead of goose quills and ink made from oak galls.

The most primitive forms of early writing were ideagraphs. Carvings on cave walls, for example, of three suns would indicate the timing of an event, such as a three day hunting expedition. American Indian tribes told elaborate stories with this method for communication.

We can trace, from archeological evidence, that the roots of our own written language began in the Near East somewhere between 3000 and 4000 B.C. This earliest communication system used approximately 200 pictures etched on clay tokens which were then counted to represent each transaction to keep records. Each clay token was incised with a symbol of wheat, oil, or whatever commodity was exchanged. After the clay was impressed these tablets were baked to form permanent records which have survived to this day.

A technological improvement was inaugurated about 3300 B.C. in Sumer. Instead of creating individual tokens for counting, the groups of pictographs were incised onto a clay surface with a wedge-shaped stylus cut from a particular plant stem. This liberated the merchants from counting piles of tokens. Gradually with their use pictures of objects became more stylized and abstract. Once they were drawn approximately the same by everybody, then universal communication was possible.

About the same time in history the Egyptians developed their hieroglyphics by carving pictures on stone to represent words in their culture. Three other world cultures independently developed pictographic writing—the Chinese, the Harappa or Mohenjo-Daro culture of the Indus valley, and the precolumbian Mesoamerican Indian culture. All other writing systems of the world, including our phonetic alphabet, were derived either directly or indirectly from one of these five through borrowing and modification.

The Chinese writing system today is basically unchanged from its original form. It is still purely pictographic. A major advantage for them is that the same pictures can represent different words, depending upon the particular dialect of each region of this vast nation. Thus they have a common written language, but not a common spoken language.

The next step in writing was a syllabary, a step toward signs representing speech sounds. Writing began to use our hearing sense, not just vision. Similar to a rebus story, for example, in English, a picture of a bee next to a picture of a leaf could represent the word, *belief.* Young Japanese children today are first taught their simple forty-syllable abstract phonetic system. Then when they enter school they begin to master the more difficult pictographs taken from the Chinese language and adapted to Japanese.

Korea also begins writing instruction with their language reduced to syllables. Charlie, in a bilingual kindergarten in California, has learned to write his name in both Korean and English. He reports that Korean is easier because it only takes three symbols, not the seven for English.

Syllable Writing

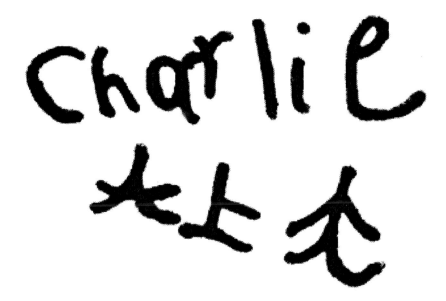

The final step in the history of writing was for each sign to stand for an individual speech sound in a particular language. The concept of a phonetic alphabet was born. An object's drawing then represented its beginning speech sound. We still do this in alphabet books (*B is for ball*). The Egyptians underwent a dramatic change evolving from their syllabic elements to twenty-four consonant signs—no vowels. This was similar to the consonantal Hebrew language today where one must supply the vowels from context.

Egyptian hieroglyphics show the beginnings of profile drawing at approximately the same time in history that they began to use their primitive phonetic communication system. It is interesting to observe that young students today, like the Egyptians, sometimes begin to draw in profile when they are beginning to use phonics for decoding skills. Beginners' profile drawings are also very similar to the early Egyptian designs in that only the head and feet are turned to the side. The body is still in a front view. One study of sex differences reports that boys usually acquire profile drawing before girls, possibly due to their need for expressing movement.

Profile Drawing

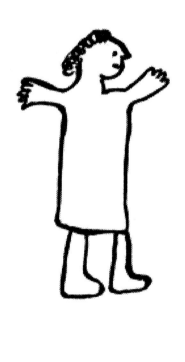
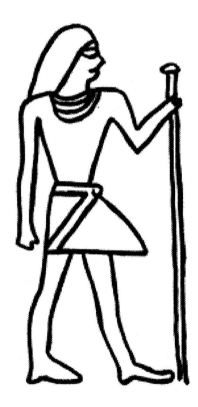

The early Egyptians, however, only used their phonetic writing system for indicating proper names, such as labels on tombstones. Perhaps the Egyptian scribes did not want to simplify their guessing game. It allowed only their priestly class to maintain its monopoly on reading and learning. With autocratic government an illiterate population is easier to control.

The Egyptian system served as a model for the Canaanite alphabet, which eventually led to the totally phonetic Greek alphabet from which all European alphabets, including our own, were later derived. Although Egyptian and Sumerian writing represent two independent systems, it is possible that as a result of commercial and diplomatic contacts, the early idea of phonetic writing was transferred from the Sumerians to the Egyptians, or vice versa. At one time experts believed that our phonetic alphabet originated in Levant (a region covering modern Syria, Israel and Lebanon) sometime after 1750 B.C. Recently, however, archeologists discovered two 18-inch stone inscriptions carved into the rock walls in a barren desert valley in southern Egypt. P. Kyle McCarter Jr., of Johns Hopkins University, an expert on the archaic alphabet, calls these the world's oldest alphabetic graffiti. With *this new discovery,* McCarter says, *now we believe that the phonetic alphabet* (with each design representing a speech sound) *was developed around 2000 B.C. by Semitic people who lived in Egypt.* Nearby these newly found signs they found Egyptian hieroglyphics which can be translated by experts in archaic languages. These indicate that the phonetic alphabetic signs were made hundreds of years before any previously recognized written alphabet.

According to McCarter, *We can recognize the letters and see how they evolved into modern forms. A letter, M, looks like the M you or I would write, only with more zigzags.* Because no other examples of this alphabet exist to serve as a key, like the Rosetta Stone, the new inscriptions cannot be completely translated. However, McCarter has identified one word as *chief* or *leader.* The carver may have left the message as a plea for safe passage through the wasteland, which was a strategic shortcut from Luxor to Thebes, across a bend in the Nile. McCarter notes that we are still in debt to those unknown innovators. *The one-sign, one-sound alphabet they devised could be learned by an adult in a few hours. It was the great revolution in human literacy.*

Oldest Known Alphabetic Graffiti

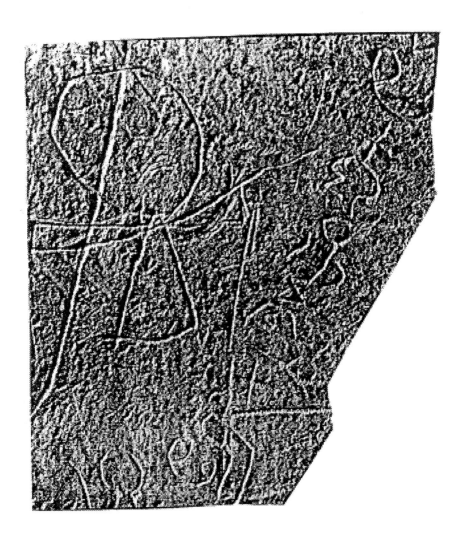

History tells us that perhaps the Seirites, a Semitic tribe living in the Sinai desert, borrowed this phonetic writing method from their Egyptian neighbor. In 1905 Sir Flinders Petrie, an archeologist, found writing there on a little sandstone sphinx in the Temple of Hathor on the site of some ancient turquoise mines. He dated the find to around 1400 B.C. This is interesting dating because it coincides exactly with the biblical period of the exodus of the Jews from Egypt.

The Sinai Sphinx

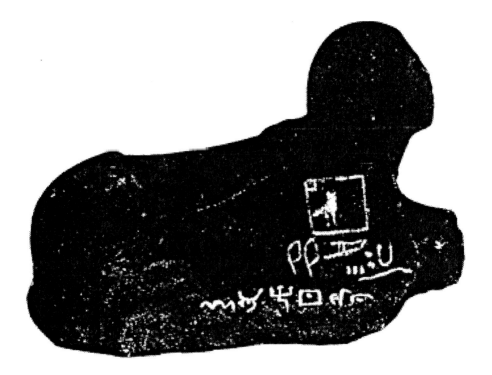

This area called, Midian, in the Sinai, is rich in copper ore. The Midianites worked the copper mines for the Egyptians. Possibly to keep records of their labors, they chose to borrow the simplest part of the Egyptian system where each picture of a familiar object represented the object's beginning speech sound. The Midianites adapted this phonetic method to their own culture and the consonant sounds of their own language.

Inscription Found in the Sinai

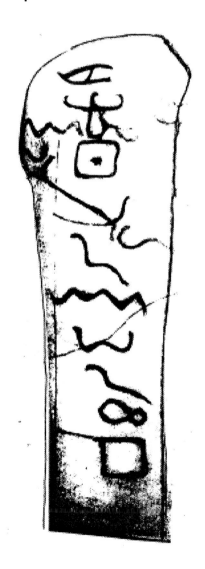

Both Christians and Jews hold that Moses brought the stone tablets with the Ten Commandments on them down from Mt. Sinai. Having grown up in the house of the Egyptian pharaoh, Moses could have been familiar with the Egyptian writing system. Also, he lived with the Midianites for a number of years and married the daughter of the Midian high priest. Moses could have learned their phonetic system from his father-in-law.

At any rate, it is assumed that the Ten Commandments were written in a phonetic alphabet with designs representing speech sounds. The concepts of monotheism (one god instead of many), codified law and a phonetic alphabet were passed on to others with Moses' Ten Commandments. It is possible that these three influenced each other. When these people were told not to worship *any graven images* did that encourage the pictographs to become more abstract?

The phonetic system of writing spread throughout the Near East, each people adapting it to their own spoken language. The Phoenicians, great sailors, carried it across the Mediterranean, first to Rhodes and Cyprus and eventually to Greece. The Greeks added four more consonant signs to cover sounds in their own language not in the Phoenician language by doubling letters (*ph, kh, ps*) and then *w,* Then they converted six unstressed Phoenician consonants into pure vowels—*heh* became *epsilon, yod* became *iota, aleph* became *alpha, het* became *eta,* and *ayin* became *omicron.* Another Phoenician sign was adapted for *upsilon.* These new symbols represented the vowel sounds we know today for our English alphabet names, A E I O U and the short vowed sound *eh.* These minor changes for the first time enabled them to accurately record every spoken word of their Greek language.

Greek Alphabet, 6th Century B.C.

ABƈD EƈCI ⊟O

IKƖ ʍʍ ⊞O--

The Greeks established a colony in Italy around 740 B.C. The Etruscans and the Romans both borrowed their alphabets from this Greek colony. The Romans transformed the Greek alphabet to serve the speech sounds of their own Latin language. As the Roman conquerors then spread throughout Western Europe, they also spread their alphabet as a common code for writing. We still use that same Roman alphabet of 26 letters, designed for Latin, and try to adapt it to our English language with 40 to 44 speech sounds.

Through the centuries each western spoken language has copied its alphabet forms all the way back to the original invention in the Near East. This system has been the model for numbers of other phonetic alphabets including English, French, Latin, Greek, Latvian, Russian, Arabic, Turkish, Persian, Hebrew and Swahili. Through a complicated process of borrowing and adaptation each culture has made changes from the original designs to fit the unique sounds of their own spoken language. In recent years there has even been an attempt to write the Chinese language in a phonetic alphabet, but it has not yet spread to wide use.

In the 1930's Dr. Frank Laubach was serving as a missionary in the primitive, remote Lanao province in the Philippines where there was universal illiteracy. He learned their spoken language and reduced it to its single speech sounds. Then he created a phonetic alphabetic system for them by using each letter as a scaffold for a simple design of a familiar object in their culture. He used the same system originated in the Near East thousands of years ago.

Dr. Laubach then taught the tribal chief to write and read with the promise that the chief then would teach the system to another. This was the beginning of his *each one teach one* basic literacy program which he spread to 103 countries using 314 languages. He was cited by UNESCO for teaching more people to write and read than anyone since the beginning of time. Today his pictographic phonetic alphabet method, adapted to our own English language, is the major form of instruction to adult illiterates in our own nation's libraries.

Laubach's Phonetic English Language System

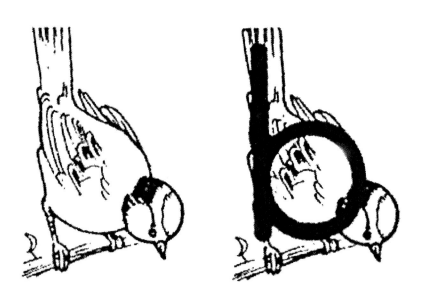

Our second letter, *B*, evolved from the Greek letter they called, *BETA*. This was derived from the Semitic word, *BET* (sometimes spelled *BETH*), which originally meant a house with four walls and was represented by a simple rectangular shape. Our English capital *B* now has two rooms and has been rounded for writing speed, but still represents the same speech sound as the first one.

The problem for English speaking youngsters today when trying to learn the alphabet letters which represent their major speech sounds is that our letters have become abstractions. The letter *B* no longer represents the beginning speech sound for our word, *house*. And the letter does not look like houses or apartments that today's children live in. Learning our phonetic alphabet is a far more difficult task today than it was in the beginning.

The Greeks used the alphabet to represent numerical order. (alpha, beta, gamma represented one, two, three). Though our letters and numerals for English are different symbols from the Greek language, we still follow that Greek *ABC* order.

The Romans gave the letters new character and elegance. Before their stone cutters incised the letters they first drew them using a brush and some kind of ink for a pattern to be followed. These flowing brush lines of the ink then were the origin of the serifs added at the beginning and ending of these letters. Roman capitals have withstood the test of time. They are still handsome, artistic forms easily distinguished from each other. When they are accidentally reversed in direction by young children, or deliberately done so by store logos, we can still read and understand them.

Classic Roman Capitals

A B C D E
F G H I J
K L N M O
P Q R S T
U V W X Y

There was no letter, Z, in the original Roman alphabet because that speech sound was not in their spoken language. It did not reappear in Latin until after the conquest of Greece by the Romans in the first century B.C. When they added Greek words to their own vocabulary such as *zephyros* (west wind) they needed the Z letter for that speech sound.

Some research tells us that capitals are easier to recognize than lower case letters. That is why so many business logos use them. But they are not easier for beginners to learn to write. They need to be written slowly because they require the ability to make right angles, to execute exact joinings of different strokes, and to make many diagonal lines. Diagonals are the most difficult writing strokes to imitate, especially for young children, because diagonals move in two directions at once, either up or down and either toward the left side or the right. There are seventeen diagonal strokes in the capital alphabet.

Here are copies of a simple horizontal diamond shape comparing samples from students age 5 1/2 and age 11. It is about 6th grade before the majority of students can satisfactorily reproduce fairly complex slanted line relationships.

Reproducing a Diamond Shape

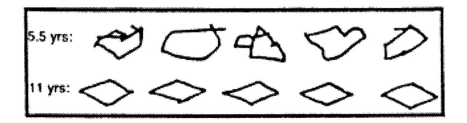

Architects and engineers today use their own specific script based on Roman capitals. Students of this profession must learn to write slowly and precisely or they would have the same illegible problem as doctors do. If their written messages were misunderstood, like doctors, then their buildings or bridges might fall down.

Architect and Engineer Script

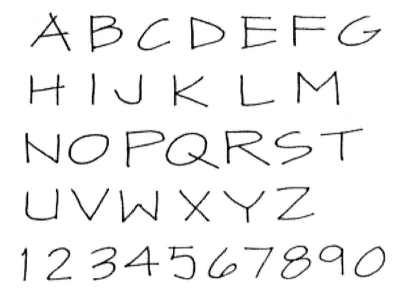

Archeological findings tell us that besides carving them slowly on stone the Romans also wrote their capital letters rapidly on slate-like material, papyrus, wax tablets and graffiti on walls. They fashioned writing tools by curing hollow reeds from the banks of the Tiber River.

Roman Capitals Written Rapidly

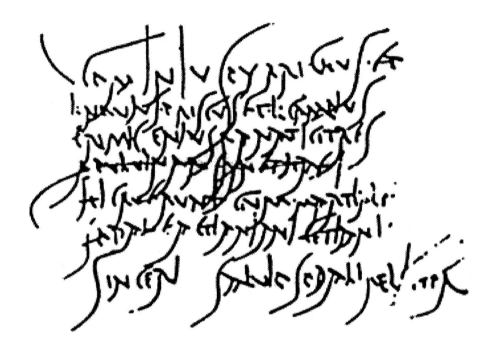

Some individuals today believe that changing their handwriting style to all capital forms will make it easier to read. This is true if they write slowly. But as soon as they write faster the separate strokes of capitals cause their writing to become hard to read. Following is an important message written in all capitals from one lawyer to another.

Rapidly Written Capitals Today

THE APPELATE COURT OF THE 9⧧ CIRCUIT HAS AGAI MADE AN EGREGIOUS DICISION AND I TRUST YOX WILL RERSE IT AND DO JUSTICE.

It certainly seems that speed of writing could also be a factor in the problem of today's illegible handwriting. Throughout history letter forms in use at various times have been beautiful, easy to read, difficult to execute, but have become scribbly and illegible when written rapidly. In addition to Roman capital letters, Roman numerals with their separate vertical and many diagonal strokes became illegible with speed. So Western Europe adopted the more free-flowing, less prone to error, Arabic numerals in the eighth century.

In the early part of the last millennium Roman letters began to take a number of alternate forms until the intervention of Charlemagne in the fourth century. He was especially interested in the study of Greek and Roman civilization and wanted this education to be spread thoughout his Holy Roman Empire, which covered a vast portion of Western Europe. Schools were almost non-existent at that time, so education was primarily in the hands of the church monasteries. There the monks carefully copied books by lettering each page by hand.

The parchment made from small animal hides on which the manuscript books were written was costly and bulky. More and more efforts were made by the monks to contract the letters to get more on a page and save materials. With the natural tendency of the hand to round corners, to leave out parts of letters and to change straight strokes into curves, each monastery invented different shorthand forms of Roman capitals in order to write them more quickly.

How Capitals Became Simplified

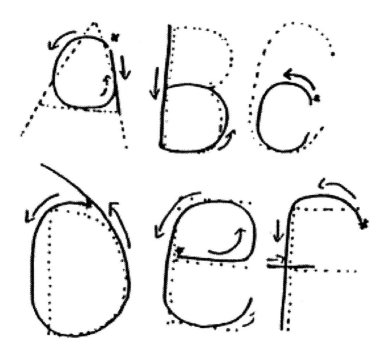

Their modified letters presented a difficulty for Charlemagne to carry out his mission because each of the monasteries in his Holy Roman Empire used their own original adaptations of Roman capitals. Monks in one area then had difficulty reading books and letters written in other monasteries in their various original script forms.

To solve his problem Charlemagne then employed Alcuin of York, a monk from Britain, who was renowned for his calligraphy. Alcuin probably received his training in Ireland because Irish monasticism and literacy were in the vanguard of Christian culture at that time.

Early Irish widespread literacy was probably due to the efforts of St. Patrick. When he was a youth in Wales, Patrick was captured by pirates and sold as a slave to an Irish farmer. Escaping one night, he fled to the Irish southern coast where he worked his way on a ship across the channel to Brittany, the north coast of France. There some monks took him in. He joined them and learned to carefully copy church manuscripts in Latin.

In the fourth century when Patrick was around thirty years old he returned to Ireland and established monasteries there to spread both religion and literacy. He introduced the Latin alphabet and its monastic variations with continuous line letters throughout Ireland to replace their primitive Celtic symbols called runes. In the dark ages following the fall of Rome these Irish monks then spread throughout Western Europe and revived literacy. An outstanding example of Irish calligraphy from over 1200 years ago can be seen today in the 600 page Book of Kells which is preserved at Trinity College in Dublin.

From the Book of Kells

abcdefz

hijklmn

opqrstu

vwxgz

Charlemagne requested Alcuin to study all the various monastery scripts used in his massive empire. Then Alcuin was instructed to choose the best elements from the scripts and construct a clear new alphabet to be used universally and which would not become illegible like rapidly written capitals. Named for Charlemagne, Alcuin's new design was called the Carolingian alphabet from Carol, the French word for Charles. Roman capitals were retained with this script only for the beginning of proper names and the beginning of sentences. Charlemagne decreed that all service books, classics, documents and other manuscripts should be rewritten in Alcuin's new form.

Eastern European countries not included in the Holy Roman Empire followed instead the alphabet directions of St.Cyril in the ninth century. These countries still use his Cyrillic alphabet, also adapted from Roman capitals, but with different forms from the Carolingian alphabet.

Alcuin's original alphabet forms gradually changed through the next few centuries to a more rapid form with elliptical shapes and a slight slope toward the right. Letters were made with fewer strokes. Sometimes some letters were joined to other letters when two adjoining strokes naturally met at the bottom or top of letters.

The quill pen was cut with an oblique point so that upstrokes came out thin and down strokes came out thick. Several Italians became especially renowned for this thick and thin calligraphy. They used flatter tops on letters which curled toward the left. Their form of letters was referred to as *italic.*

In the sixteenth century Alcuin's alphabet forms were commonly used for church correspondence and this style was named *chancery cursive.* The term, *cursive,* meant that all letters were made with a rounded continuous line, path or course. Not all letters in each word were joined.

Chancery Cursive

the quick brown
fox jumps over
the lazy dog

This is the form used by Queen Elizabeth I (1558-1603). Historical records show us that she was a highly intelligent and thoroughly educated executive of that period. She used the chancery cursive form for official and personal correspondence.

Later, in the Baroque period of art, the late 16th, 17th and early 18th centuries, fancy decorations and flourishes became popular for all art forms and affected handwriting. At this time copy books to teach handwriting were engraved on copper plates so they could be reproduced by stamping on a surface rather than having each page hand-lettered. Each Baroque engraver outdid each other with more curly lines and extra flourishes. It was easier for the engravers to keep their tool, called a *burin*, on the surface rather than lifting between letters. So they swirled a line up to the beginning of each letter and all letters in each word began to be joined. For the same reason jewelers today also usually join letters when engraving.

At this time metal pens replaced quills and handwriting became an art form, called *roundhand* or *copperplate*, because it imitated engraving. Obviously this elaborate form would become illegible if written rapidly. Our Declaration of Independence was written in this art form.

Copperplate Cursive Capitals

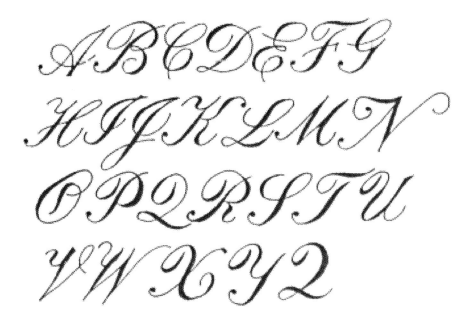

Copperplate Lower Case

abcdefghijklm
nopqrstuvwxyz

In the nineteenth and twentieth centuries publishers of handwriting materials for schools removed some of the flourishes, but kept the engravers' joining strokes. They also kept the elaborate baroque capitals. This is the form of copperplate cursive writing usually still taught in a number of American schools today, beginning about third grade. When drawn slowly it is an art form. When written quickly it becomes illegible. It does not fit our computer age. It is the major cause of medical mistakes.

Standard School Cursive

abcdefghijklm
nopqrstuvwxyz

In the early part of the twentieth century students were expected to exe-cute this copperplate cursive alphabet with a metal tip pen and liquid ink in a bottle. School desks were designed with a hole in the upper right cor-ner for the ink bottle. The pen was pointed with a long ink slit which often snagged on the upstrokes, especially with rough school paper. This caused frustrated students to make unsightly blots and ink splashes.

In 1922 Marjorie Wise, a British graduate student, came to the United States to study American education. For her thesis at Columbia University she produced a short teacher manual entitled, *On the Technique of Manuscript Writing*. To conform to the available copperplate metal pen, Wise suggested that a handwriting program for beginning writers should make lower case letters with separate strokes as in Roman capitals. Each letter should then be made with only down strokes to prevent ink splashes on rough school paper. Preliminary drill on letter strokes would be unnec-essary with this simple form.

Wise emphasized that students should not attempt to model their writing on *anything as uniform and characterless as printing*. Each person's writing instead should express the individuality of the writer. She intended that students should continue her simple models into mature life-long fluent writing rather than change in upper primary grades to copperplate cursive forms. Her manual suggested that such easy writing would gradually develop into a natural joined manuscript without the flourishes of copperplate.

Some teachers misinterpreted Wise's message and began to use a more rigid and geometric form of letters with round circles and vertical lines they called *manuscript* or *ball stick*. Although Marjorie Wise was effective in launching manuscript writing for beginners she rejected her work in 1924 as ill-advised and misused. She said this form was too slow and it caused young children to make reversals of letters. This was especially true of those made with circles and adjoining vertical lines (*b, d, p, q*) when young children have not yet developed sufficient laterality to distinguish left and right sides for objects outside the body.

Wise recommended instead going back to the italic variations of the old chancery cursive originally created by Alcuin with each letter made with continuous lines instead of written with separate strokes. Wise was a charter member of the British Society of Italic Handwriting.

In spite of Wise's objections, ball stick manuscript writing forms acquired professional credibility associated with Columbia University. Her rejection was too late. By 1924 American publishers had already jumped on the band wagon. In two years they had already spent considerable funds to develop and distribute copy books, teacher manuals and wall charts (those white letters on dark green from your school days). The publishers believed that their investment was too great for them to change again to the continuous line forms now recommended by Wise.

Consequently, after 76 years, in spite of Wise's admission of error, these ball stick manuscript letter forms are still commonly taught to beginners in the early primary classes of many American schools. And they are the most common form of letters on American toys and workbooks purchased by preschools and parents of young children today.

Ball Stick Manuscript

a b c d e f
g h i j k
l m n o p
q r s t u
v w x y z

Just as primary level students are beginning to develop fluency with these circle and vertical stick manuscript letter forms (about third grade) the majority of American schools today switch back to the 19th century copperplate cursive form with ovals and slanted lines. Letters are then expected to begin with an ascending stroke, as if we were engraving them. All letters in each word are expected to be joined. Fancy loops are added for all ascending and descending strokes with extra flourishes from the Baroque period. Eleven of the capital letters (those underlined) have little resemblance to the Roman forms students see in print.

School Cursive Capitals

The disadvantages of this commonly taught school cursive are many. The absence of pen lifts by joining each letter in a word cramps the hand and tires the beginner. This cursive form needs full-arm motion which is not feasible today for quick writing on sales slips, checks, clip boards carried by paramedics, notes from an instructor or on medical prescriptions. When written rapidly the loops flatten out and this form becomes scribble. Also, if the hand could travel through the air some of the time and just join letters which naturally slide into each other, instead of joining all the letters in each word, more time and energy could be saved.

American adults whose handwriting becomes illegible when written quickly (especially physicians) are victims of our culture which continues to teach two archaic forms of handwriting, ball stick manuscript and copperplate cursive. Neither of them fits today's world. We are no longer locked into the narrow range of movement required by writing with the copperplate metal pen designed long ago. A pseudo artistic system is still taught to American students instead of a durable, simple, legible handwriting model for every day use with today's more versatile writing tools.

CAN WE CHANGE?

The Food and Drug Administration is taking some steps to alleviate errors in prescriptions. They are looking for software that can screen potential new names for drugs against the 10,000 brand names and 7,700 generics in use today in North America. One such system is now in place that sets names for new generics. It has been suggested that doctors note each patient's illness on the prescription form. Some hospitals now enter prescriptions by computer and put a bar code on pill bottles. One company, called, *Allscript*, has developed a handheld computer so doctors can avoid handwriting.

These moves would solve only prescription errors, not hospital and operation mix-ups, and not the thousands of dollars lost each year by industries and merchants because of illegible handwriting. Will it become more of a worldwide problem now with the continuing spread of English? As Asian children learn English as a second language, what form of alphabet will they be taught? Will it be the same separate stroke ball stick manuscript and archaic copperplate cursive, which cause so many communication problems here?

Adults, including parents and teachers, cannot assume that young students who exhibit handwriting difficulties will automatically improve as they mature. It is obvious when we view adult's handwriting that this is a false premise. Students' handwriting will deteriorate, as the school's demands increase and become more complex in both time and space. Some students will avoid the act of writing whenever possible.

Later, when they are free from teachers' demands that they write in the archaic copperplate cursive, a number of courageous adolescents and young adults express their independence and invent their own handwriting systems. They join only those letters whose strokes naturally touch as they slide toward the right. These individuals eliminate unnecessary strokes at the beginning of letters and avoid loops for ascenders and descenders. They are reinventing Alcuin's chancery cursive forms. This modified form has become so commonly used that now there is a computer font for it.

Today's Reinvented Chancery Cursive

Our season passes at Donner
aren't doing us much good
this week. We seem to be
experiencing a snow drought

Modified Cursive Written on a Computer

We are about to have our first home. Our yard, our porch. Neighbors and people passing by stop and watch in awe.

Writing today needs to be produced in contexts where people are under pressure to get things done quickly—to draft reports, business letters and manuscripts, and to write examinations and applications for employment. Computers and word processors are an enormous aid today to both presentation and production, but they have not eliminated the need for simple, legible, fluent handwriting. Similarly, the spell-check component is available on computers, but that does not eliminate the need for teaching students to spell.

One attempt to change how we teach handwriting to American students was made by Donald Neal Thurber when he was teaching first grade in Michigan in the mid 60's. He said that when he was showing his young students how to write with vertical strokes and round circles in ball stick manuscript it suddenly occurred to him that in two more years they would be expected to write with the slanted lines and ovals of copperplate cursive. Their discontinuous stroke practice in first grade would have to change to a flowing rhythm. He then began to teach beginners each letter made with a continuous line. After three years his alphabet spread to other teachers and was launched by a major publisher in 1978. They named it D'Nealian by combining the author's first two names.

D'Nealian Lower Case

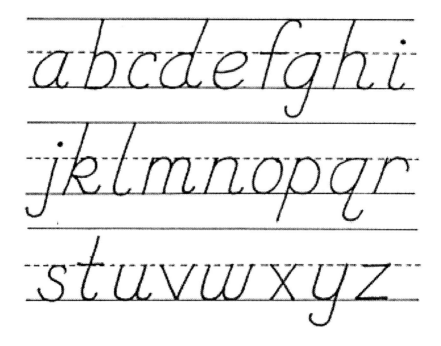

    Some American schools have changed from ball stick manuscript to D'Nealian for beginners. Making each letter with a continuous line is certainly a step in the right direction. But the advantage is lost when young beginners are expected to add joining strokes at the end of letters.

    Thurber has a patent on these strokes he calls *monkey tails*. Thurber's handwriting system was invented for his first grade students, usually at least six years old. However, letter formation today is often introduced in American kindergartens when students are usually only five or less.

At that age a number of young children often lack the necessary neurological control to execute the joining strokes of this design correctly. Five year olds usually cannot stop their upward swing of the D'Nealian joining strokes. Each letter then looks like it is followed by a letter, *U*. In addition, immature perception at this age causes beginners to sometimes confuse the added joining strokes on both lower case *t* and *l* with the bottom curve on the letter, *j*.

However, these are minor compared to the major problem with D'Nealian. The published form of this system recommends a switch in about third grade to the old copperplate cursive intended for engraving in the Baroque period. At that time the engravers' swirls at the beginning of each letter and loops for ascenders and descenders are added. We know when we look at adult's handwriting that when written rapidly copperplate cursive becomes illegible. The D'Nealian published program makes one step forward and two steps backward.

D'Nealian Cursive

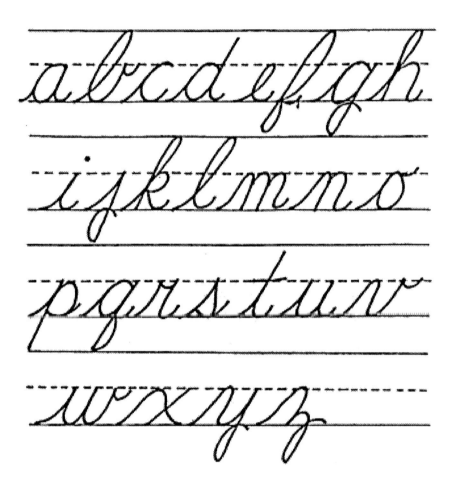

Thurber, himself, who is now a retired teacher and principal believes that conventional copperplate cursive taught by elementary teachers today, including his own published program, is simply an arbitrary benchmark for literacy at the third grade level. He is quoted in a recent edition of a Canadian magazine. *Everything in the business world, in the real world,*

is either typed or printed. So why use cursive at all? If the goal is the passing of information back and forth, it should be done in the most legible fashion, not the most illegible one which is conventional cursive.

Another move to change school handwriting instruction was made in Oregon in the last century. After extensive trials in the area around the city of Portland with italic forms recommended by Marjorie Wise back in 1924 the state of Oregon officially adopted the italic letter system as one of four programs that schools could use.

Some handwriting programs tell young students to begin alphabet letters which aim toward the left side to start at (*the two o'clock position on the clock*). In today's world of digital clocks a number of school beginners are not familiar with the face on a traditional clock. Also, when they begin left curve letters at this place their right hand covers the stroke. Some young beginners then reverse the stroke so that they can see what they are doing. One major advantage of the italic form for letters is that their beginning strokes for these letters (*a c d g q*) start instead with a horizontal line toward the left instead of a curve. This helps to prevent the reversals of some beginners.

Italic forms are based on the ellipse shape which is more natural than the circle shape of ball stick. The major advantage of the italic form is that it can be used for life. Students do not need to change from one form to another as they proceed from grade to grade. Early instruction starts with simple, continuous-line forms.

Italic Lower Case

abcdefghij

klmnop

qrstuvwxyz

With increased fluency italic writers gradually make natural joinings of letters which bump into each other as they write words toward the right side. Roman capitals blend well with italic when needed for beginnings of names and sentences. Another advantage of italic is that it usually does not become illegible when written rapidly like the loops and flourishes of the copperplate cursive form.

Italic Written Rapidly

Here is an example of
Italic Handwriting
written quickly.

Another individual option with italic could be to use Alcuin's old Chancery capitals with it.

Chancery Capitals

ABCDEFGHIJ

KLMNOPQ

RSTUVWXYZ

The Australian education system originally followed our same American system using ball stick manuscript forms for beginners and the copperplate cursive form beginning in late primary years. Their system caused the same medical mistakes by their physicians, pharmacists and other health care professionals, as we are experiencing today. In order to overcome their problem they made a major change in handwriting instruction in their schools.

About 15 years ago they adopted a system of continuous line letters to be used for all ages. Their students do not change in mid-stream to a different form. Unlike italic, however, the Australian letters, *k, w* and *y*, are made with rounded forms, rather than the more difficult and slower diagonal lines of italic. The swirls up to the beginning of each letter originally added by engravers on copper plate and the loopy ascenders and descenders which cause illegibility with speed have been eliminated. Like the italic system, Roman capitals are used with this new Australian form for beginnings of names and sentences.

Notice that instead of introducing these letters in traditional *ABC* order they are first taught to beginners in-groups with similar shapes. Also, to prevent reversals by young children with undeveloped lateral direction, letters which are oriented toward the left side are taught in a different group from those which aim toward the right.

Australian Lower Case

l t i u y j

a d g q c o e

n m h b p k r

f s v w x z

In an attempt to determine mathematically which of the alphabet let-terforms usually taught in American schools would be the easiest for young beginning writers to acquire, I devised a difficulty scale with seven factors. The first factor refers to the Beery research which determines at what age specific strokes appear in children's scribbles and drawings from age 1 to 6. The decimal represents months of age–2.10 represents 2 years ten months.

Beery-Butenika Scale

|	2.10	□	4.6
—	3.0	\	4.7
◯	3.0	✕	4.11
✛	4.1	△	5.3
╱	4.4	‹	5.6

Alphabet Difficulty Scale

1. MATURATION OF STROKES according to the sequence of strokes which appear in children's scribbles and drawings from age 2 to 6.

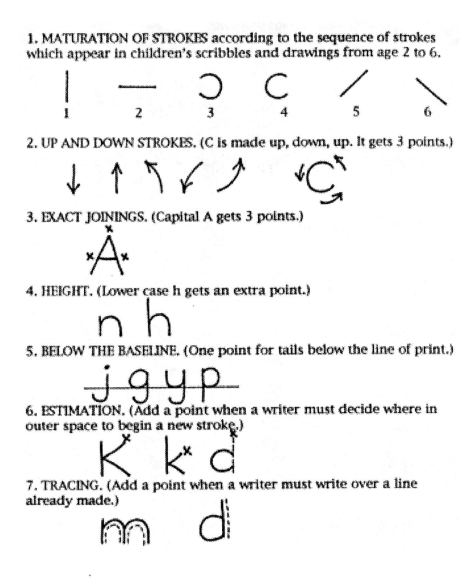

2. UP AND DOWN STROKES. (C is made up, down, up. It gets 3 points.)

3. EXACT JOININGS. (Capital A gets 3 points.)

4. HEIGHT. (Lower case h gets an extra point.)

5. BELOW THE BASELINE. (One point for tails below the line of print.)

6. ESTIMATION. (Add a point when a writer must decide where in outer space to begin a new stroke.)

7. TRACING. (Add a point when a writer must write over a line already made.)

To demonstrate the difficulty scale, capital *A* scores 5 points for the left diagonal stroke, 6 points for the right diagonal, 2 points for two down strokes, 2 points for the horizontal line, 1 point for the direction of the horizontal line, and 3 exact joinings of strokes, or a total score of 19 points. Capital *A* is one of the most difficult alphabet letters for beginners to make. Unfortunately it is also the most common letter which unaware parents and teachers try to teach first to young children because it is first in the *ABC sequence.*

Using the difficulty scale and a calculator, all 26 capitals sum to 322 points. Among the lower case forms, ball stick manuscript sums to 278, italic sums to 272, and D'Nealian to 247. The Australian form sums to only 237. Obviously all these commonly used lower case forms are easier to write than capitals. If the *monkey tails* for the letters a, *d, h, i, l, m, n,* and *t* in D'Nealian are not taught to beginners this form would score even less in difficulty. Then to further prevent reversals of letters by beginners we can add the flat tops of italic for left curves *a, c, d, g,* and *q.* Such a beginners alphabet would add to only 244 points.

Capital Letter Difficulty

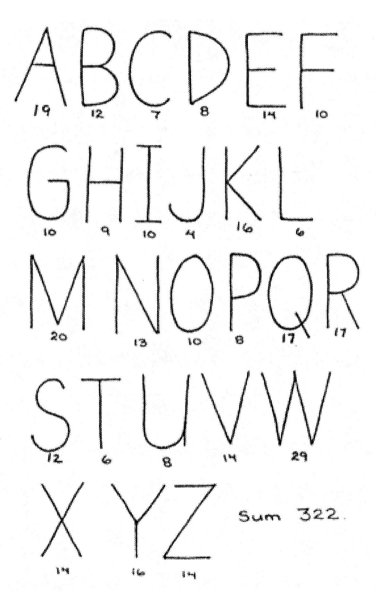

Sum 322.

Ball Stick Difficulty

a b c d e f g
11 10 7 11 12 7 11

h i j k l m
7 3 6 12 5 10

n o p q r s
7 10 10 18 5 12

t u v w x y z
7 8 14 29 14 15 14

Sum 278

Italic Difficulty

a b c d e f g h i
11 9 8 13 8 8 13 7 3

j k l m n o p q
6 10 5 12 7 10 11 14

r s t u v w x y z
6 12 8 7 14 29 14 9 14

Sum 272

D'Nealian Difficulty

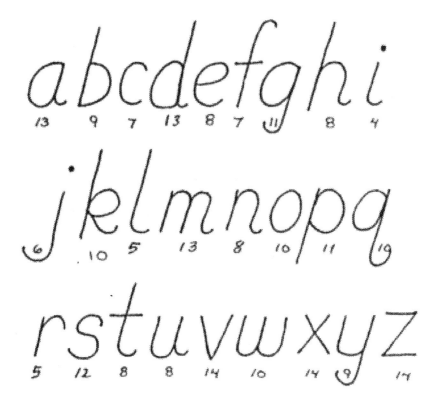

Sum 247

Australian Difficulty

l t i u y j
3 7 3 8 9 6

a d g a c o e
12 11 11 10 7 10 8

n m h b p k r
6 12 7 9 11 16 5

f s v w x z
7 12 9 10 14 14

Sum 237

Simplified Lower Case (monkey tails Removed, italic flat tops added)

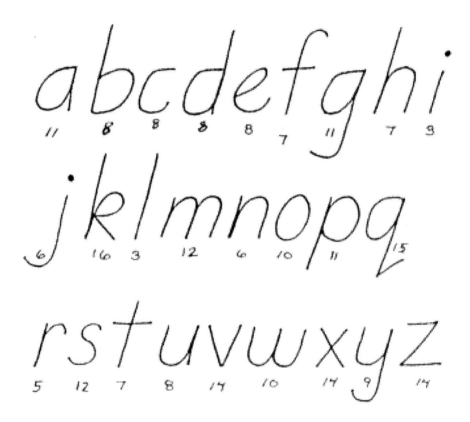

Sum 244

This simplest form can be practiced by beginners in shape groups like Australian forms in which the initial strokes are the same or aim at either the left or the right side. Notice that the least difficult letters to make are first. The letters, *t, l, and i* can usually be made by a two or three year old child. The left curves are separated from the right curves to help prevent reversals. Those with diagonal strokes, the most difficult, are taught last.

Like the Australian alphabet and the italic alphabet, this simplified lower case form can be used for life. When written rapidly letters in which the last stroke is on the right side will naturally join the following letter. Those letters in which the last stroke ends on the left side will not join. Students will not need to learn a second form of handwriting. There are no loops. There are no ascending curves at the beginning of letters. This easy to write form can be written rapidly and still maintain legibility.

Simplified Letters Grouped by Shape

l l l l	i t l j
ccc	c a d f g o s e q
mm	r n m p b h k
ww	u w y
ЛЛЛ	v x z

Simplest Form in Continuous Communication

When you write in this modern chancery cursive letters naturally join if the upswing toward the right touches the beginning of the following letter. Unnecessary loops, swirls and joinings are not added. Roman capitals blend well with it. An extra set of capital letters does not need to be learned.

To lessen the gap in opportunity between higher income families and those with minimum finances, some politicians are promoting universal preschool for three and four year olds. If this comes to be, then some people probably will be expecting these youngsters to begin to write alphabet letters. Let us hope they will choose one of the easier letter forms, not ball stick manuscript or capitals.

For generations the Japanese have been successfully expecting their three-year-olds to happily draw, write and read over forty abstract syllable symbols before entrance to kindergarten. They used to do it with black ink and a paintbrush. Children would make the ink by scraping a solid bar of ink and then mixing the residue with water. This mud-pie like activity was supposed to strengthen the muscles in their fingers and wrists for writing. Today black markers, less messy, are probably taking over and possibly wipe-off white boards.

This draw-write skill, with young children copying meaningful symbols of Japanese culture, usually takes place in the home under parent supervision. A child, for example, could learn to make the three symbols for *TO, YO*, and *TA* then tell you he or she has made the name for the family car, a *TOYOTA*. Picture books for preschoolers are available in this simple phonetic system so that they can follow up writing these syllables with learning to read them. Japanese educators claim that their culture produces few dyslexics.

Japanese Language Symbols for Beginners

ア A	イ I	ウ U	エ E	オ O
カ KA	キ KI	ク KU	ケ KE	コ KO
サ SA	シ SHI	ス SU	セ SE	ソ SO
タ TA	チ CHI	ツ TSU	テ TE	ト TO
ナ NA	ニ NI	ヌ NU	ネ NE	ノ NO
ハ HA	ヒ HI	フ HU	ヘ HE	ホ HO
マ MA	ミ MI	ム MU	メ ME	モ MO
ヤ YA		ユ YU		ヨ YO
ラ RA	リ RI	ル RU	レ RE	ロ RO
ワ WA		ン N		ヲ O

Standing at an easel, white board or paper taped to a wall for early scribbling and drawing, rather than sitting at a table or desk takes advantage of natural gravity. This establishes the habit of making lines going from top to bottom, so important for later fluency in writing English in any of the suggested forms for beginners. Also, a smooth sliding black marker on a light colored surface will enhance visual perception necessary for later reading.

Nicolas, Age 3, Makes Vertical Lines

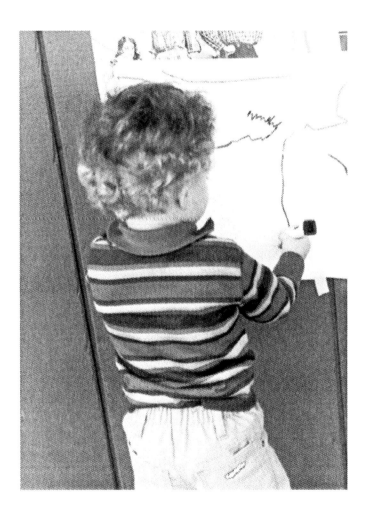

Like the Japanese, British cultures throughout the world also assume that parents will accept the responsibility for teaching their preschoolers basic alphabet skills (both letter formation and simple phonics) before entrance to school. New Zealand children enter school on their fifth birthday whenever it occurs throughout the school year. While visiting their schools at any time during the year the newcomers can be pointed out by their teachers. On their first day in what they call *entry level* (our kindergarten) most New Zealand beginners will independently write (not copy) one or two original sentences in their journals. This writing activity lays a strong foundation for reading instruction which will follow in that entry-level year. American students are usually not expected to read until first grade.

Writing before reading was strongly suggested in Italy in the beginning years of the 20th century. At that time in Rome, in the Industrial Revolution, farmers had come into the city to work in the new factories. Both parents worked as well as most teen-agers. Alone, with no supervision, packs of young children were destroying property. Dr. Maria Montessori was sent there to save the public housing. First she showed the children how to care for their surroundings. Then she created games to teach them basic academic skills. In her journal she wrote about her surprising discovery. *Show young children how to write and they will then spontaneously explode into reading.* Another journal entry she shared from her experience reads, *Writing is easier than reading because children know what they have written. In reading they have to discover the thoughts of others.*

Carol Chomsky, of Harvard Education Department, also recommends that students begin literacy education with the skills for writing independent messages (both phonics and letter formation) before they are expected to read.

Could it be that this practice of expecting young children to write before they are expected to read might have some effect on preventing or alleviating dyslexia? Brain research during the last twenty or more years at the University of California at Berkeley and two studies, one at Harvard, and a more recent one at Yale, suggest this possibility.

We used to think that intelligence was fixed at birth. Now brain research has shown us that the active human brain is constantly growing and changing, especially in the preschool years. Four-footed animals are born with a much more mature brain than the newborn human brain. The newborn giraffe, for example, must stand within minutes after birth and run with the herd or be a tasty lunch for hungry lions. On the other hand, the newborn human's brain is much less mature. It takes about one year of growth before that brain can control walking.

It is a matter of engineering. The female animal which walks on two legs, such as kangaroo or human, must have a very thick and strong pelvis to support the individual in an upright position. It then takes a smaller head and brain to pass through the smaller birth canal in the upright pelvis. Growth in the brain after birth then needs to be stimulated by individual sensory experiences in the early years encouraged by parents or other caregivers. We were shocked not too long ago by the news of the number of Rumanian orphans who were being physically, mentally and socially retarded by being stockpiled alone for months in cribs with propped bottles for feeding.

In both the Harvard and the Yale study students who were labeled dyslexic were hooked up to a computer which then showed the part of the brain which was active for specific different activities. In the Yale study when given reading tasks the brains of these students were overactive in the frontal areas, especially the area for producing speech instead of the area which links letters to sounds in sequence to form words.

It is a task in direction. English writing goes from left to right, then returns to the left side of the next line of print. The Harvard study showed strong deficiency in the rear part of the brain controlling direction of movement. Students in the study were confused on *Which Way* questions. Could it be that frequent early drawing and early writing, moving lines in specific directions, could activate this part of the brain necessary for reading? Could it be that the Japanese and British cultures are on the right track for beginning literacy with expecting writing before reading to enhance direction?

Does writing before reading incur a gender factor? In a summary at Stanford University of 1400 research studies of sex differences in learning basic academic skills only one difference showed up. These studies show strong evidence of a sex-linked gene that contributes to spatial ability. Approximately 50 percent of boys have it, but only 25 percent of girls. Writing is a spatial act. This study indicates that boys in general have a stronger innate capacity to learn to write than girls. In the United States, however, we usually have more boys than girls in remedial reading groups. Could it be that teaching writing before reading might lessen the number of boys needing special help?

How soon should we start? One youngster of my acquaintance began in his high chair. When he was happily smearing pudding, making patterns on the tray like finger painting, his mother gave him an alternate activity. She taped a paper to the tray and gave him a black non-toxic marker for scribbling. After a few scribble sessions he realized he had control of the tool and his marks became less random and more deliberate. Scribbling became one of his favorite daily activities. By age two he had developed the neurological control to stop his spirals and make a rough round shape. Instead of praising his making a picture of a *wheel or balloon*, his mother told him he had made a picture of a noise he makes with his mouth, an *ah*. She took him to a mirror and showed him that when he opened his mouth widely his lips formed a circle as he made this noise. Was she pushing phonics on a toddler instead of waiting till he was of school age? Or was she just helping him become more aware of his own voice noises at the time of life when he was acquiring speech? Is this not the time when the fast growing young human brain is richest and most active in discriminating sounds?

The most common speech sound representing the letter, *O, in* English, is *ah*, as in *ON*. At any rate Tyler was delighted in this discovery and continued to make more round figures and saying *ah*. Then he found more of them on license plates, signs, the newspaper and in his picture books.

His scribblings and drawings were celebrated and hung for all to see. When he accidentally made more letter shapes he was told the major sound in English representing these shapes. Eventually he had acquired enough letters and the speech sounds they represent in English to write his own words. At age four he could not read or spell yet, but he learned through scribble play to listen to the sounds of his own speech and happily record anything he could say with the forms of a simple alphabet.

Tyler's Grocery List, Age 4

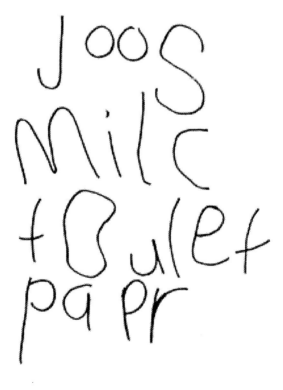

Tyler's Halloween Costume, Age 5

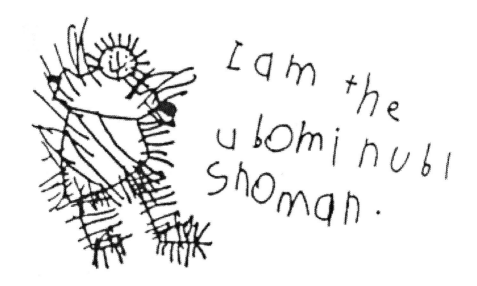

If Tyler's preschool or kindergarten teacher had expected him to spell English conventionally like the dictionary, he probably would have lost interest in writing. In his first grade he was still writing enthusiastically and spelling by ear. Following is his science report at age six:

Tyler's Science Report

Buterflys and moths have a hed a thorax and a abdomen. In ther blud tha have diferent culers. I saw that wen it was squishd. Moths have feelers that look like fethers.

> Puterflys have
> nobs on top of ther
> feelers. Moths fly
> at nite but not
> buterflys. A thick
> body is a moth. A thin
> body is a buterfly.

Tyler's independent science report has 59 words. Using his ear for language he has spelled 44 of them in the conventional English patterns found in a dictionary. He discovered through his scribble and drawing play that the alphabet is a phonetic code to record language sounds, a system which was invented over 3000 years ago.

Before English was frozen into type with the invention of the printing press, the same word was often spelled in a variety of ways. In Queen Elizabeth's time it was considered to be especially literate and creative to deliberately vary the spelling of words in the same piece of writing. Shakespeare did it often, even with his own name.

Sam, one of my kindergarten students, was an early reader who had discovered that our printed language used a variety of ways to represent speech sounds. He was not yet aware that eventually he would be expected to write them according to our English dictionary. He knew how to write *fat*, but he preferred to write it *phat*. He played his spelling game at the painting easel. First he drew a face and head with a crown on it. Under his drawing he made four columns, each headed with one of the letters representing the four sounds in the word he heard when he said, *queen* (k, oo, ee, n). Then he listed all the possible ways he knew how to write the four sounds. Finally he put them together to make twelve different ways to phonetically spell and write the word, *queen.*

Spelling conventional English is the most difficult of our language arts. Einstein once said that spelling English is the hardest task that mankind has ever imposed on itself. Yet he preferred to write in English rather than in his native German because he could be more precise with our language which has so many words. It has been said that *English spelling was concocted by Anglo Saxon storytellers, French scribes, and Dutch printers using an Italian alphabet.*

The major reason for our spelling's difficulty is that the first books printed in English around 1476 were designed by Dutch typesetters who could neither speak nor write English. They had no rules for setting up type in a language foreign to them. So they made up their own rules. They transposed English words beginning with *hw* to *wh.* In English these words were pronounced with a definite expulsion of air at the beginning, represented by the letter, *h.* The Dutch and German forms of these words, more familiar to the typesetters, begin with a *w.* So they respelled the question words such as, *hwen* to *when* and *hwat* to *what.* Then they added a *w* letter to *who.*

These inventive Dutch compositors also used the French pattern, *le,* instead of the Anglo Saxon *el* for ending syllables. So they changed words like *appel* to *apple* and the former *lytel* to *little.* They changed the former simple spellings of the words *feld, yeld and sege,* to the Germanic *ie* pattern more familiar to them, resulting in *field, yield* and *siege.* Then they even used the same pattern changing *frend* to *friend* though it has a different vowel sound from the others.

The consistency of spelling was much less important to them than their graphically pleasing even margins. If a compositor needed an extra letter to even out a margin, he usually selected the letter most easily reached. Directly in front of him in the type case was the place for the letter, *e.* This is probably the source for the unnecessary *e* on the end of *there, where,* and *were.* Before the first dictionary these words had no final *e.* The word, *hus,* for a dwelling was pronounced *hoos.* These *Dutchmen* changed it to the more familiar French spelling pattern, *hous,* as in *soup.* Then they added an *e.* All these bizarre spellings invented by the original Dutch compositors are now frozen into type and considered correct. Thousands of words have been added to our dictionaries since then. Today we are expected to spell them according to the same patterns invented by those first typesetters rather than according to their pronunciation in English.

Consequently, conventional English spelling is so difficult that it should probably be postponed until children are reading about middle first grade and are confidently composing and writing what they hear. Then they usually notice that the most frequent English words they see in their reading, the, *to, of, was,* etc. are not spelled the way they sound. One follow-up research study tells us that young children who spell first by ear, like Tyler, will be superior spellers by the fifth grade, *providing they have been later taught and expected to learn the basic rules, patterns and generalizations of our written language, not just expected to memorize a list of words.* If schools skip this most important step in elementary and secondary levels, students will spell by ear forever.

This six-year-old has already learned some basic spelling rules. She is on her way to becoming a good speller if she continues to learn the rules.

Emily's Story

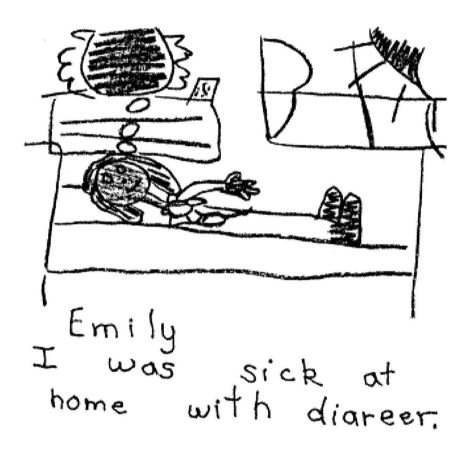

Emily should get full credit for—a capital at the beginning, a period at the end, the *ck* at the end after a short vowel, the final *e* letter and the double *e* pattern to indicate long vowel sounds, the correct symbols for all the speech sounds in her story, spelling memory for the frequent English word, *was*, and attempting to spell *diarrhea* phonetically and meaningfully. When she can read about third grade level she will have the skills to look up difficult spellings in a dictionary.

Tyler lost his pleasure and excitement about writing in his second grade when the primary grades at his school adopted a new composition program. With this new system the children dictated sentences to the teacher who wrote them on the wall chalkboard. When their story was complete all the students were then expected to copy it on paper. This copying task is especially difficult for young children when the immature muscles of their eyes have to change back and forth from far vision to near vision and back again. Also, white marks on a dark chalkboard are difficult to see, like the negative of a photograph. Today's white boards with wipe-off pens are far superior.

Copying is no more than visual exercise. The child is not learning to write his talk. He or she is being alienated from his own sounds and speech rhythms. It puts the emphasis on mechanics–on periods, capitalizations, identations instead of on communication.

In Tyler's third grade he was expected to change his easy to read and easy to write letterforms for archaic copperplate cursive. His handwriting became totally illegible. Fortunately his family owned a computer for his high school assignments. Today he makes a good living as a computer specialist, but his writing requires a slow translation. Following is a sample.

Tyler's Signature

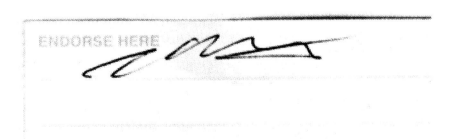

In addition to teaching simpler alphabet forms than ball stick manuscript and chancery cursive and starting writing in the early years, what other changes might be made to help reduce the numbers of medical mistakes and mishaps?

Could schools change their traditional curriculum? We know that the currently taught copperplate cursive is one of the major factors in medical mistakes. This form cannot be written rapidly and maintain legibility. Written slowly it is an art form. Our fast-paced lives do not afford that luxury today. Instead of requiring all upper primary students to use the archaic copperplate cursive form it could be offered as an elective in upper grades as an art form called *Calligraphy.* Such a name would give it status. Or students could be taught how to read archaic copperplate cursive as a special writing code used by their ancestors, but not expected to write it.

Could state standards change? Most educators tend to resist change. California's State Board of Education, however, seems to be aware that a change is needed. In their newest *Standards for Language Arts they* do not stipulate which writing forms to teach in grades 1 and 2. They also give teachers a choice for handwriting forms in the third grade. That standard reads, *write legibly in cursive or joined italic, adhering to margins and correct spacing between letters in a word and words in a sentence.* Copperplate cursive writing alone is thus not required in that state. It will be interesting to see if legible handwriting will be included in their new state test under construction.

Could adults (including physicians or medical students) relearn to write in any of the modified cursive forms with each letter made with a continuous line and which eliminate the archaic engravers' loops and flourishes? The Australians have shown us how. Any of these forms can be written quickly without distortion. All it would take for change is a bit of effort and commitment.

This is the same as retraining one's physical memory to perfect a golf swing, improve one's skill at tennis or any other sport, or learn the movements to play a musical instrument. Modified cursive handwriting forms could even be offered as an elective course in medical school.

Handwriting is not merely mechanical movement as if the people who produce it are simply made of levers, springs or pulleys. It depends on manual control to an extent. Being able to see helps. But the important organization goes on in the brain. It takes time for the brain to send a message to the fingers, instructing them to produce a set of movements and then to receive the message about what has been done. Before the message gets back, the brain has sent out the next message. The brain is ahead of the fingers. The writer must integrate the auditory, visual and motor systems in order to complete this complex skill.

In writing, like playing a musical instrument, the body creates what neurophysiologists call a ballistic movement. This requires the initial electrical burst, lasting just long enough to get the muscles moving at the right speed and in the right direction. A ballistic movement relies on only one signal. Its trajectory, force and speed have to be just right, and carefully worked out in advance. Then the brain is free to think about the next movement. And, like music, practice is the key to success.

Notice how you hold your writing tool. For efficiency and fluency it should be held between the middle finger, index finger and thumb. Only the index finger is placed on top of the tool, about one-inch above the point. This grasp is the most efficient and will be the least tiring for the muscles of the fingers and hand. This is the same grasp that those knowledgeable about etiquette insist is correct for holding a fork or spoon for eating.

If kindergarten and first grade children are still holding a spoon or fork in the fist like a weapon they will have a most difficult time learning to hold a writing tool efficiently. Parents and teachers can show them how to balance the tool on the middle finger and the first joint of the pointer finger for eating. Simply turn the wrist down for writing.

Efficient Grasp of Writing Tool

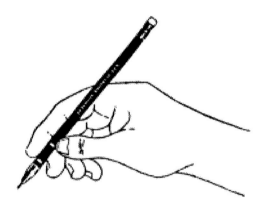

Calvin of the comics is six years old but still uses the very primitive infant's tool grip. Miss Wormwood, his first grade teacher, will have a difficult time trying to change Calvin's inefficient habit so he can learn to write with fluency.

Primitive Infantile Tool Grip

Calvin and Hobbes   **by Bill Watterson**

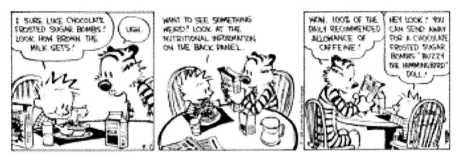

No two writers will have the same handwriting. A statistician determined that the possibility of two writings being identical is one chance in 68 trillion. Adults should develop their own individual writing, but at the same time they need to keep in mind that writing is for communication. It must be easily read by one's self and others. Fluency is influenced by body position and furniture. In recent years a rash of individuals have developed wrist, back and neck problems from strained positions at their computers. The same is true for prolonged sessions of handwriting. It is tiring for the neck and shoulders if you have to raise your arms for writing. So sit high enough so your elbows can rest on the tabletop. Use a pillow if necessary to give you height. A small stool under your feet will prevent lower back fatigue.

Notice that Calvin's table top is at his chest level. That is why he has to raise his whole arms. Miss Wormwood needs to ask the school administration for school furniture in different sizes to fit different children. This is especially necessary at ages six and seven when some children have already acquired the individual, natural spurt at that time in the growth of the body's long bones in arms and legs.

Writing with the left hand takes more energy than the right because letters must be pushed across the paper rather than pulled by the right hand. Notice that Calvin is eating with his left hand. Poor Miss Wormwood! She needs to show Calvin how to tilt his paper so it is parallel to his writing arm. If you are a lefty, tilt yours far enough so you can easily see your writing to prevent hooking the wrist.

Paper Position for Lefties

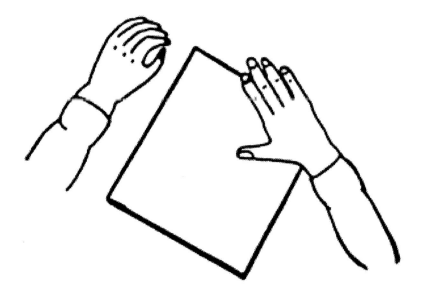

Writing fluency is also affected by the nature of the writing implement. Handwriting began to make a serious downhill curve with the invention of the ballpoint pen in around 1940. Ballpoint lines are fuzzy and tend to smear. Adults who are serious about improving their handwriting need to look for pens which make a firm, clear line. The handwriting models at the end of this book's appendix were made with a fine felt-tip marker. Also, a calligraphy pen with an oblique tip seems to improve the appearance of everyone's handwriting.

Young children should never be given a number two pencil. It is so hard that they have to firmly push it onto the paper to make marks that they can see. This is tiring for the hand and wrist muscles and causes inefficient grasp of the tool. Look for number four pencils which make a dark line with little pressure. For very young children cut the pencils in half so they are crayon size. We don't give them a full size scissors. Why expect them to write with an adult size pencil? With supervision, let them draw and write with fine line felt tip pens. Black, of course, is best for enhancing visual perception. After their drawings are finished they may add color.

Scientific language is full of words based on Latin and Greek such as *ontogeny recapitulates phylogeny.* This phrase reminds us that the growing human fetus in the womb takes similar steps that humankind took in development. Similarly, young children go through the same steps in learning to write as historical and archeological records show us how civilization developed writing.

First they begin with the pictograph stage. When a child independently draws a humanoid and names it this is a very important milestone. Such a drawing, with just a closed line and adjoining rays for limbs and possibly dots for eyes, shows that the child has developed the hand-eye coordination to begin to learn to write lower case letters—not capitals with their many difficult diagonal lines. Many of these lower case letters are made with these same strokes, a closed line shape with adjoining rays. Secondly, when the child spontaneously names the figure, *That's Daddy,* or some other significant person, you know that the child is mentally ready to begin to learn other abstractions such as alphabet letters. An abstraction is something that represents something else. A two-year old demonstrates the dawning of abstraction when she offers you a wooden block and tells you it is a cooky.

The following child's drawing also shows two letters, *D* and *M.* She shares, *My picture story says, Dani is my mom.* Her letters represent whole words, as in early Egyptian hieroglyphics.

Kaci's Picture Story

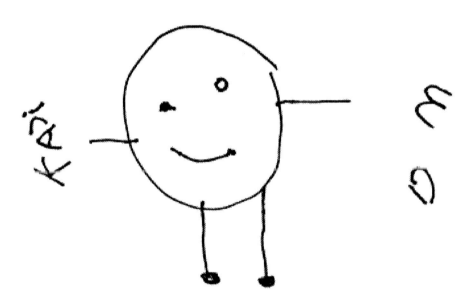

In the history of writing development a syllabary was the next step when a drawing represented just part of a word. When children learn the names of alphabet letters before they learn the speech sounds they represent they sometimes use letters for whole syllables or even whole words. When his busy mother was not listening to him this preschool child wrote her a note. The first two letters are whole words. His letter, f, represents the syllable, *ef.*

Paul Uses Letters as Words and Syllables

RUDF

The Greek culture was first to develop a complete phonetic alphabetic system to cover all the consonant and vowel sounds of their language. This child is repeating history as a true writer because she can listen to her own speech and record anything she can say. Now she has the important skills for learning to read. She can reverse the task from encoding to decoding. As Dr. Maria Montessori told us over 80 years ago, she will probably spontaneously *explode into reading* with little formal instruction.

Krista's Picture Story

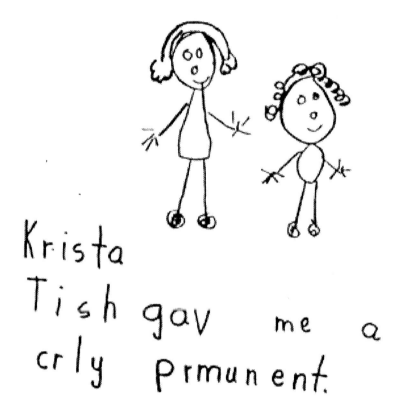

Krista
Tish gav me a
crly Prmunent.

CONCLUSION

In 1956 two organizations, the International Council for the Improvement of Reading Instruction and the National Association for Remedial Teaching merged and became the International Reading Association (IRA). According to its bylaws this organization has three goals—*to improve the quality of reading instruction at all levels, to develop an awareness of the impact of reading on the citizenry,* and *to sponsor conferences and meetings planned to implement these purposes.* These are all laudable goals.

Most of the concern about literacy today is focused on teaching reading. This financial interest is sponsored by the IRA whose leaders are the authors of school reading programs and the hundreds of book publishers who naturally want to push their wares. They have been very successful in convincing parents of the very important task of purchasing books to read with their young children. To further their own interests they have convinced the public that reading is the most important school skill.

There is no comparable lobby for teaching writing. No one agitates for the improvement of writing instruction or seeks to impress our citizens with writing's importance or calls conferences or meetings to advance these two objectives. There is no international writing association, no national writing association and no regional, state, county or school district writing association. Reading experts have convinced administrators and teachers that reading instruction is the all-important study of their professional careers.

The Council for Basic Education continues their story, *Go Back to Basics*. Basics to them means reading and math. Ford and Carnegie have spent thousands and thousands of dollars for reading research but not one cent for early writing research.

No one in history is remembered and eulogized because he or she was a great reader. Today, a well-written application with a legible signature for a job or for acceptance to one's first choice of a college may get you in. A long list of books you have read won't do it.

This push for reading at the expense of writing is primarily economic. As they say in Washington, *It's the economy, STUPID!* There is little monetary profit in materials for teaching handwriting which requires no books. A good salesperson expects to earn thousands of dollars selling books. He or she won't make it selling pencils and paper.

Surfing the internet for handwriting information turns up only a number of authors who claim to be specialists in handwriting analysis—*to give you a personality test, to learn how to determine the identity of a criminal with forensic analysis,* and even *how handwriting can change your life.*

But there is little current research on how to teach handwriting. This would be fertile ground for a graduate thesis. A 300-page book, published late in 1999, entitled *Interactive Writing*, discusses in depth how to teach composition to children in the kindergarten, first and second grades. The extensive bibliography for this book lists 69 authors of 92 research studies on writing. Obviously young students also need to learn how to form alphabet letters in order to participate in these composition activities. But there is no mention in this book about how to teach handwriting to young children.

A 1998 edition of a Canadian magazine has an article entitled, *Penmanship, What's That?* There is an interview with Professor Beyestein of Simon Fraser University in Vancouver. He agrees that handwriting is a problem with the young adults he teaches. *It seems that there are more illegible workbooks coming across my desk these days.*

Kate Gladstone, who is a specialist in handwriting teaching in Albany, New York, is also interviewed for this article. She says that today's communication needs are primarily met with e-mail, word processing on the computer and telephone calls. But Gladstone believes *that handwriting must be taught because there is probably more handwriting done now than 15 years ago, because of the fax machine where many documents are annotated by hand before transmission.*

To summarize, the December, 1999, shocking report warns us that 98,000 Americans die every year because of medical mistakes. The evidence shows that the major cause of these deaths is faulty misinterpreting of doctors' orders by pharmacists, hospital attendants and other medical personnel.

When individuals become doctors they take an oath that they will harm no one. There is one simple way we can help the next generation of doctors live up to their oath and stop these unnecessary medical accidents and deaths. We can stop requiring the teaching of two archaic forms of alphabet, ball stick manuscript and copperplate cursive, in both our public and private schools. We know that these two out-of-date forms cannot be written rapidly and still retain legibility.

Secondly, let us think about the written communication skills that future doctors will need. Perhaps we should begin earlier with younger children to lay foundation skills for handwriting like the Japanese and British cultures do. It takes about two years for toddlers to express themselves in meaningful oral communication. Should we not also give young children two years to learn to express themselves in handwritten communication instead of waiting and then trying to jam it into the first six weeks of first grade when they are also expected to begin to learn to read?

If we teach alphabet skills to younger children we need to keep in mind what Jerome Bruner, an educational psychologist and one of the original architects of HEAD START, reminded us, *It's not WHAT you teach, but HOW you do it that makes for success.* These alphabet skills can be imparted to young children through developmentally appropriate activities: scribbling, drawing, clay modeling, manipulative activities, stories and dramatic play–all dealing with simple alphabet forms. Perhaps the most important activity is encouraging youngsters to make marks on a surface. As soon as they have the dexterity to hold and use a spoon they also can manipulate a writing tool.

One interesting evidence of the power of our phonetic alphabet when taught with developmentally appropriate ways concerned an autisic six-year-old who was mainstreamed into a kindergarten class. He had receptive language, but his only spoken language was counting to ten and naming both upper and lower case alphabet letters. When asked a simple question such as, *Would you like a drink of water?,* he would throw himself onto the floor in a screaming tantrum, which is the typical frustration behavior of autism without speech.

His kindergarten teacher was using a phonetic alphabet program which was similar to how Frank Laubach successfully taught illiterate peoples throughout the world by imposing pictures directly onto alphabet letters. The children were told stories about letter-animals which made particular noises (not alphabet letter names). This is the same mental level as expecting toddlers to respond to animal picture books when we ask them, *What does the cow say?* We expect, *MOOO.*

Next the children were shown how to draw the skeleton of each animal in the story (an alphabet letter). Then they were directly shown how to draw six more strokes turning each letter into the animal making the noise in the story. The children added a *talking balloon* in comic style with a letter inside, then repeated the noise of the letter-animal in the story. Eventually the students were expected to associate the letter and its major speech sound without the picture addition.

The autistic child thrived on this method to teach the correspondence between letters and speech sounds with this simple drawing approach. He acquired the speech sounds he had missed as an infant and toddler. Miraculously he then put his sounds together into spoken syllables and words and exploded into spoken language. Usually we expect children to talk before they can write and read. This child did it in reverse.

As Montessori showed us over 89 years ago, he then exploded into reading. At eight years old he could read at the fifth grade level. At fourteen today he still sometimes acts a bit aloof. But he is literate and can hold up his end of a simple conversation. He is successful in school and without doubt he will eventually be able to function successfully as an independent adult.

Like the Australians who faced their problem and corrected it, we can replace our commonly taught writing forms in American schools with one of the alternative modified cursive alphabets without the curls and swirls of copperplate cursive. These simple forms can be taught to young children, They do not become illegible with rapid writing and can be used for life. It is time to stop wringing our hands about medical mistakes, look at the obvious cause, and do something about it!

Today, with the invention of the most powerful weapons ever conceived by man, we are in danger of destroying the earth. The most reasonable defense against such a catastrophe is for all peoples to develop an understanding and respect for each other's culture. Only a small fraction of people in the world have the opportunity to visit each other to develop this knowledge. It is possible, however, to transmit this information through writing and reading. Dr. Frank Laubach showed us how to do it back in the 1930's. He saw literacy as a means of filling empty stomachs and preparing minds for self-rule. Universal literacy, both writing and reading, therefore, needs to be a world priority.

The invention of the phonetic alphabetic system thousands of years ago was a gigantic step toward civilization as we know it today. It has been said that this invention was even more important than the invention of the wheel. It has been adapted to express most of the world's written languages. It is the major tool for continuing civilization as we know it. We need to respect and celebrate this invention by giving emphasis to these modified cursive letter forms which were originally developed by Alcuin in the eighth century. They can be written quickly without distortion.

It is time to stop blaming doctors for these unnecessary deaths caused by miscommunication. The fault lies instead in our national education system which continues to teach the archaic handwriting forms developed to engrave on copper over 300 years ago which do not fit today's needs and which are the major cause of thousands of deadly medical mistakes.

BIBLIOGRAPHY

The related problems of medical mistakes and handwriting are not new. These references are listed in reverse chronological order from the years 2000 to 1926.

Dawn of the ABC's. New York, NY: Discover, March, 2000.

Clinton wants hospitals to report deadly mistakes, Associated Press, February 22, 2000.

*Problem Prescriptions,*Des Moines,IO: Consumer Reports, January, 2000.

McCarter,Andrea. *Interactive Writing.* Portsmouth, N.H.: Heinemann, 2000.

Pear, Robert. *VA Medical Mistakes, 700 dead in two years.* San Francisco CA.: San Francisco Examiner, December 19, 1999.

Ouaknin, Marc-Alain. *Mysteries of the Alphabet.* New York, London, Paris: Abbeville Press Publishers, 1999.

Medical Errors Called Major U.S. Killer. San Francisco, CA.: San Francisco Chronicle, November 30, 1999.

Kantrowitz, Barbara and Anne Underwood. *Dyslexia and the New Science of Reading* :Newsweek, November 22, 1999.

Diamond, Marian. *Magic Trees of the Mind.* New York: Dutton, 1998.

Gladstone, Kate. *Penmanship, What's That ?* Alberta Canada: Alberta Report Newsmagazine, Volume 25, Issue 19, April 27, 1998.

Cahill, Thomas. *How the Irish Saved Civilization.* New York: Doubleday, 1995.

Chomsky, Carol. *Writing Before Reading Eighty Years Later,* in Loeffler, *Montessori in Contemporary American Culture.* Portsmouth, N.J.: Heinemann, 1992

Connell, Donna Reid. *Writing is Child's Play.* Napa, CA.: Addison-Wesley, 1995, Can Do Books, 1999.

————————*Integrated Total Language, (itl).* Napa, CA.: Can Do Books, 1999.

————————*STAGES-Sequential Tasks to Assist the Growth of English Spelling.* East Aurora, N.Y.: D.O.K. Publishers, 1989. Napa. CA.: Can Do Books, 1995.

Literate Doctors. San Francisco, CA · San Francisco Chronicle, March 26, 1989.

Beery, Keith. *Revised Test of Visual Motor Integration.* Cleveland, Toronto: Modern Curriculum Press, 1989

New Med School Exam Seeks Doctors Who Can Write, San Francisco CA.: San Francisco Chronicle, March 14, 1989.

Clay, Marie. *Writing Begins at Home.* Auckland, New Zealand: Heinemann, 1987.

Doctors Are Risking Death by Abbreviation, San Francisco CA,: San Francisco Chronicle, December 27, 1987.

Logan, Robert K. *The Alphabet Effect.* New York: William Morrow and Co., 1986.

Read, Charles. *Children's Creative Spelling. London:* Routledge and Kegan-Paul, 1986.

Logan, Robert K.. *The Alphabet Effect.* New York: William Morrow and Co., 1986.

Graves, Donald. *Write From the Start.* NewYork: American Library, 1985.

Connell, Donna Reid. *Writing Before Reading.* ERIC, ED 260 423, April, 1985.

——————————*Handwriting, Taking a Look at the Alternatives.* Novato, CA.: Academic Therapy, 1983.

Thurber, Donald Neal. *Write On! With Continuous Stroke Print.* Novato, CA.: Academic Therapy, 1983.

McKean, Kevin. *Beaming New Light on the Brain.* New York: Discover 2, December, 1981.

Nelms, Henning. *Thinking With a Pencil.* Berkeley, CA.: Ten Speed Press, 1981.

Harries, Rhonda and Mildred Yost. *Elements of Handwriting.* Novato, CA.: Academic Therapy Publications, 1981.

Two Kids Get the Wrong Operations. San Francisco CA.: San Francisco Chronicle, June 7, 1980.

Amend, Karen and Mary S. Ruiz. *Handwriting Analysis.* Hollywood, CA.: Newcastle Publishing Co. 1980.

Ibuka, M.. *Kindergarten Is too Late.* New York: Simon and Schuster, 1980.

Bissex, G.L.. *GNYS AT WRK, A child learns to write and read.* Cambridge, MA.: Harvard University Press 1980.

Briem, Gunnlaugur. *Teaching and Learning the Craft of Handwriting.* Visible Language, Volume 13, No.1, 1979.

Gray, Nicolette. *Towards a New Handwriting Adapted to the Ball-point Pen.* Visible Language 13, 1979.

Thurber, Donald Neal. *D'Nealian Handwriting.* Glenview, IL.: Scott Foresman Publishing 1978.

Wellington, Irene. *The Irene Wellington Copy Book.* New York: Pentalic Corporation, 1977.

Fischer, John H.. *Chancery and the Emergence of Standard Written English in the Fifteenth Century.* Speculum, 1977.

Lehman, Charles. *Handwriting Models for Schools.* Portland, OR.: Alcuin Press, 1976.

Read, Charles. *Lessons to be Learned from the Preschool Orthographer.* Foundations of Language Development. New York: Academic Press, 1975.

Connell, Donna Reid. *The Insertion of Writing Skills into Kindergarten Curriculum.* Urbana, IL.: ERIC Clearing House on Reading and Communication Skills, as ED 260413, 1975.

Maccoby, Eleanor, *The Psychology of Sex Differences,* Palo Alto, CA.: Stanford University Press. 1974.

Scragg, D.C., *A History of English Spelling,* New York :Row, 1974.

Chomsky, Carol. *Invented Spelling in First Grade.* Buffalo, N.Y.: Paper presented at Reading Research Symposium, State University of New York 1974.

Lehman, Charles. *Simple Italic Handwriting.* New York: Pentalic Corporation, 1973.

DiLeo, Joseph. *Children's Drawings as Diagnostic Aids,* New York: Brunner/Mazel Inc., 1973.

Eager, Fred. *Guide to Italic Handwriting,* Caledonia, New York: Italimuse, Inc. 1970.

Bruner, Jerome S.. *The Relevance of Education,* New York: W.W. Norton, 1971.

Eager, Fred. *The Story of Handwriting and a Fresh Solution.* Grand Island, N.Y.: Italic News, 1970.

Reimer, George. *How They Murdered the Second R.* New York: W.W. Norton 1969.

George, Ross. *Speedball Textbook.* Hunt Manufacturing Co., 1965.

Gelb, I.J. *A Study of Writing,* Chicago and London: University of Chicago Press 1952.

The Hippocratic Oath. Supplement to the History *of Medicine*, Text, Translation and Interpretation by permission of the Johns Hopkins University Press, 1943.

Connard, Edith. *The Growth of Manuscript Writing in the United States.* Childhood Education, January, 1935.

Goodenough, F.L.. *Measurement of Intelligence by Drawings.* New York: World Book Co., 1926.

ABOUT THE AUTHOR

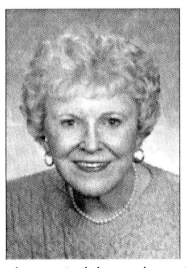

Dr.Connell's first career was as a journalist. Her byline, Donna Reid, in a west coast magazine was lifted by an agent who was seeking a stage name for a fledgling actress.

Donna's other claim to fame was inventing the hole in Cheerios during her advertising role. After W.W.II she and her husband moved to a rural area to raise their four young children in a safe, tranquil environment. This led to an egg business with 3000 cooperating hens. Their neighbor was the school superintendent who recruited them to be teachers, though neither of them had experience in the field.

Donna acquired that know-how as teacher-principal of a one-room school. Later she applied the one-room attributes by pioneering multi-age grouping and parent aides at a larger school which became the model for the state's early childhood program. Her favorite activity is showing young children how to compose and write their own original thoughts. Then, to everyone's surprise, they explode spontaneously into reading. Today she serves as a consultant for that write-to-read approach to beginning literacy.

APPENDIX

Your Mysterious Prescription

If you can understand your doctor's prescription you might be able to check to see if the pharmacist has filled it correctly. If you had any Latin instruction in the long ago past, see if you can supply the Latin words for these abbreviations.

ODE	MEANING
Rx	Latin for Recipe (Take)
aa	of each
gtt.	a drop
pil.	pill
caps.	capsule
s	without
c	with
b.i.n.	2 times a night
t.i.n.	2 times a day
t.i.d.	3 times a day
q.i.d.	4 times a day
q.4h	every 4 hours
q.s.	as much as is required
ad lib	as desired
p.r.n.	when required
stat	immediately
s.o.s.	if necessary

gm.	gram
o.d.	every day
p.c.	after meals
a.c.	before meals

Suggestions for Improving Your Handwriting

If you are seriously trying to make your handwriting easier to read, pay particular attention to these letters (t, e, a, r, n, o and d). Extensive research has proved that these seven letters cause the most illegibilities. Malformations of the letters a, r and t are estimated to account for 45 percent of unreadable alphabet letters. Also, watch out for these:

INTENDED LETTER	LOOKS LIKE
a	u,o,or ci
b	li
d	cl
e	i
i	e
h	li
k	u
m	w
n	u
o	a
r	i or n
t	l
w	m or ur

Don't mix capitals and lower case letters. Notice the difference between Ff, Jj, Kk, Ll,Pp and Yy. Join only letters which naturally bump into each other. A letter, p, does not join because it ends on the left side. In addition to the classic sentence which uses all 26 letters,

The quick brown fox jumps over the lazy dog, here are some other choices for practice. Can you invent your own original sentence with all 26?

William said that every-
thing about his jacket
was in quite good con-
dition except for the
zipper.

As we explored the gulf in Zanzibar we quickly moved closer to the jutting rocks.

Venerable Will played jazz sax til 3 o'clock in the morning before he quit.

Joe was pleased with our gift of quail, mink, zebra and clever oryx.

Traveling beneath the azure sky in our jolly ox-cart, we often hit bumps quite hard.

Alfredo just must bring very exciting news to the plaza quickly.

Anxious Al waved back his pa from the zinc quarry just sighted.

- A complete kit for teaching handwriting and phonics as foundation skills for beginning reading.

- Teaches letters as pictures of noisy animals, similar to Laubach's highly successful world-wide picture-letter program for adults.

    - Plus Writing is Childs Play, a 127 page explicit parent-teacher guide telling WHY, WHAT and HOW to enhance these important literacy skills.

Send for BOTH itl and the guide for 75.00, plus shipping

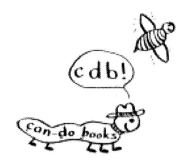

2119 Lone Oak Avenue
Napa, CA., 94558
707-224-0197